Tini Treesa Benny
K Sathya Narayanan

DENTAL FLUOROSIS

Tini Treesa Benny
K Sathya Narayanan

DENTAL FLUOROSIS

MANAGEMENT DENTAL FLUOROSIS

LAP LAMBERT Academic Publishing

Cover image: www.ingimage.com

Publisher:
LAP LAMBERT Academic Publishing
is a trademark of
Dodo Books Indian Ocean Ltd. and OmniScriptum S.R.L publishing group

120 High Road, East Finchley, London, N2 9ED, United Kingdom
Str. Armeneasca 28/1, office 1, Chisinau MD-2012, Republic of Moldova, Europe
Managing Directors: Ieva Konstantinova, Victoria Ursu
info@omniscriptum.com

Printed at: see last page
ISBN: 978-620-8-44165-4

DENTAL FLUOROSIS AND ITS MANAGEMENT

INTRODUCTION

Fluoride is a naturally occurring mineral. It is a member of the halogen family with an atomic weight of 19 and an atomic number of 9. The word Fluorine is a Latin derivation of "Fluore" which means "to flow". In rock and soil, Fluorine occurs in combination with a variety of minerals such as Fluorspar (CaF_2), Fluoroapatite ($Ca_{10}(PO_4)O_6F_2$) and Cryolite (Na_3AlF_6). Out of which Fluorspar is the principle fluoride containing mineral with a content of 49%. [1]In dentistry, the use of fluoride is considered to be an important factor in the prevention and management of dental caries. Dental caries is one of the major dental diseases affecting a large population worldwide. It affects the quality of life by causing pain and discomfort and placing a huge financial burden on public health services. [1]

Fluoride prevents dental cavities by promoting remineralization and preventing demineralization at the crystal surfaces inside the tooth. This is due to the fluoroapatite crystals that grow on the surface of the tooth, which are extremely resistant to acid attack by the bacteria. It is also well known that fluoride destroys the bacterial enzymes necessary for glucose metabolism. If fluoride consumption occurs during the early stages of tooth formation, it may result in surface (sub-surface) hypomineralization. In addition to aqueous solutions, fluorides can also be administered topically as gels, pastes, foam, varnishes, rinses, etc. [2] Fluoridation of milk, salt, and water can all be used to deliver systemic fluorides. Community water fluoridation has shown to be the most successful of these, particularly for schoolchildren.[3] fluoride controls caries lesion development, primarily through its topical effect on de and remineralization processes taking place at the interface between the tooth surface and the oral fluids. This concept was established after very elegant in situ studies described by *Øgaard et al.*[4] When fluoride was first introduced in caries prevention, water fluoridation was followed by a decline in caries, while interruptions in fluoridation were followed by increasing caries levels. However, the recent decades have shown significant caries decrease even though there was poor water fluoridation. The authors proposed that one of the reasons might be the availability of other fluoride-containing products, e.g. fluoride dentifrices.[5] The results of more recent epidemiological and laboratory studies can be summarized by stating that post-eruptive (topical) application of fluoride plays the dominant role in caries prevention.[6] However, this concept does not discount the effectiveness of systemic fluoridation methods. Recent studies indicate that fluoride in drinking water has a beneficial pre-eruptive effect on caries prevention. Using fluoridated water before tooth eruption is more effective than using it only from eruption until age 15, particularly in protecting all surfaces of the first molars, with the most significant impact seen in pits and fissures. [7]Dental fluorosis is a developmental disturbance of dental enamel, caused by successive exposures to high concentrations of fluoride during tooth development, leading to enamel with lower mineral content and increased porosity.[8] The excessive consumption or inhalation of fluoride causes skeletal fluorosis. It results in skeletal abnormalities. This condition is chronic, caused by prolonged ingestion of high concentrations of fluoride, although acutely high levels of fluoride may cause death through intoxication

Dr. Fredrick Mckay's arrival in Colorado Springs, Colorado, USA, in 1901 marked the beginning of everything. He saw a specific, seemingly permanent stain known in the area as the "Colorado stain" in all of the patients there. They conducted investigations on people living in different communities in various parts of the Country. After discussing this issue with *Dr. G.V. Black* in 1916, and they came to the conclusion that a "unidentified agent" was to blame for the stain and mottled enamel. They assumed that this component was present in the water these people drank while their teeth were calcifying. *Churchill H.V.*, a chemist, provided more confirmation of this in 1931 when he discovered fluoride in water via spectrographic analysis. Fluoride was therefore discovered to be the "mystery component" behind the Colorado stain after thirty years. Foods and beverages derived from fluoride-containing soils as well as fluoridated water can all contribute to fluorosis.[9]

Dental fluorosis is a disorder of dental enamel formation brought on by repeated exposure to high fluoride concentrations when teeth are developing, resulting in enamel with lower mineral content and increased porosity. It has been suggested that similar fluoride doses may result in different levels of dental fluorosis.[8] Because the severity of dental fluorosis depends on when and for how long the overexposure to fluoride occurs, the individual response, weight, level of physical activity, nutritional factors, and bone growth.

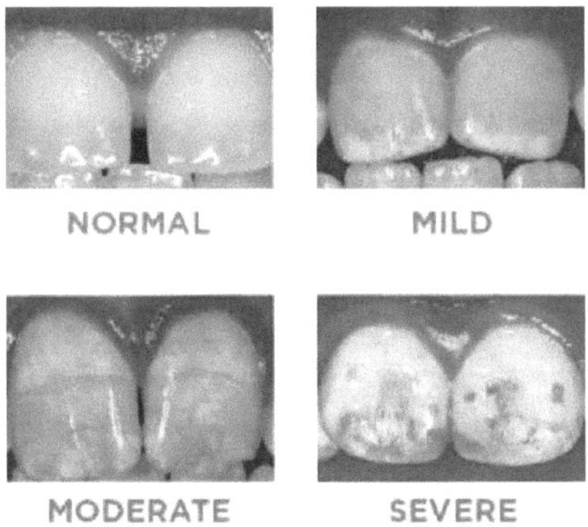

Fig 1: Types of dental fluorosis (source: Fluorosis Facts: Information Parents & Caregivers - HealthyChildren.org)

Due to enhanced perikymata, opaque white lines may be visible. The white lines may confluence in some circumstances while remaining distinct white opaque zones in others. The clinical characteristics change as the illness becomes more severe. In more extreme situations, the entire enamel surface may appear chalky white and may become extremely porous. After eruption, the sub-surface porosity may draw extrinsic stains, causing enamel pitting and tooth discoloration. [10]

Fluoride levels in the plasma are connected to how severe fluorosis is. Many factors, such as total fluoride intake, method of intake (inhaled or swallowed), renal function, pace of bone metabolism, metabolic activity, etc., affect plasma fluoride levels in the body. The degree of enamel fluorosis has also been demonstrated to be influenced by genetic factors in addition to these other variables.[11]The maximum concentration of fluoride in drinking water that the WHO recommends is 1.5 mg/l. [12] Due to the presence of excessive fluoride in groundwater, the World Health

Organization (WHO) lowered the permissible limit of fluoride in drinking water in India from 1.5 to 1.0 parts per million (ppm) in 1998 (UNICEF 1999). The reason fluoride contamination often goes unnoticed is that fluoride does not affect the color, taste, or odor of water. Therefore, individuals consuming fluoride-contaminated water often become aware of the issue only after experiencing symptoms of fluoride-related diseases. Fluoride toxicity in humans can lead to various symptoms, including stained teeth, skeletal fluorosis (a bone disease that causes paralysis and deformities such as stooped backs, crooked hands, and legs), blindness, and other physical abnormalities. In areas where fluoride contamination is prevalent, the impact goes beyond just health issues and becomes a socio-economic problem. (12)

Despite the United Nations declaring the "Decade of Water for Life" from 2005 to 2015, many people still lack access to safe drinking water. To address this problem, solutions are necessary to alleviate the suffering of those without access to safe drinking water and individuals affected by fluoride-induced diseases. However, effective mitigation can only occur once the areas potentially affected by fluoride contamination are accurately identified, delineated, and mapped. This mapping process is crucial for targeting interventions, implementing water treatment measures, and ensuring that affected communities receive the necessary support and resources to overcome this issue. (13)

Aesthetic alterations in dental fluorosis are the main cause of worry. Between the ages of 20 and 30 months, children are more susceptible to this issue if they are exposed to fluoride in excess. Between the ages of one and four, fluoride overexposure is most dangerous. By the age of eight, this decreases considerably. The youngster may experience psychological repercussions as a result of having low self-esteem. Fluoride ingestion is safe within a daily range of 0.05–0.07 mg F/kg. (8) The main cause of endemic dental fluorosis is fluoride in drinking water exceeding 1.5 mg/L.(12) Moreover, incidences of fluorosis linked to toothpaste, fluoride supplements, infant formula, and seafood consumption have been documented. Several tissues and systems have also been impacted by persistent fluoride exposure. However, between 4 and 8 ppm can cause the bone to grow dense, and between 8 ppm and 10 years of exposure can cause crippling osteosclerosis.[14]

The clinical appearance of dental fluorosis has been characterized by several criteria. The first three are frequently employed. They include the Dean's index, the Thylstrup and Fejerskov index, and the fluorosis index of the tooth surface. More recently, the Fluorosis Risk Index (FRI) has been in use.[9] Many different types of treatments have been tried throughout history. According to *McCloskey,* the first attempt to eliminate fluorosis stains was carried out by *Dr. Walker Kane*, Colorado Springs, in 1916. He used muriatic acid to scrub his teeth. He first used the flame of an alcohol torch to hasten the acid's entry into the enamel and dentin. He heated the teeth with a warmed instrument before applying the acid. [15] Bleaching has been suggested for the fluorosis cases that are the least severe. Enamel micro abrasion and whitening are two clinical therapies for moderate dental fluorosis. Composite restorations combined with enamel micro-abrasion or the placement of attractive veneers can be used to treat severe stains. For more severe cases, prosthetic crowns might be necessary. More importantly, dentists should inform parents about food choices, particularly those that indirectly contribute to dental fluorosis, like infant formula, meals, and sodas that require water to make.[8]

The treatment options available to improve the esthetics affected by fluorosis are based on the severity of fluorosis. In reference to TF index, various treatment options include noninvasive and minimal-invasive methods. Noninvasive methods include removing the surface stained areas through teeth bleaching, using micro-abrasion techniques, combination approaches, and using ACP-CPP technology while invasive approaches include using veneers, laminates, or crowns. These techniques have shown varying degrees of success and have been used with different protocols. Among the noninvasive methods, bleaching with H_2O_2, or carbamide peroxide has been considered the least invasive approach and has been successfully used in children and adolescents. In addition to these, recently resin infiltration, a technique originally advocated for arresting early caries and for esthetic management of white opacities associated with early caries, has also been reported to treat fluorosis stains. The rationale for using resin infiltration for fluorosis stains is that these lesions resemble white spot demineralization. Both involve subsurface hypomineralization beneath a relatively well-mineralized surface, which allows for effective infiltration with resin.[16]

HISTORY

In 1901, a dentist named *Frederick McKay* in Colorado, USA, observed that many of his patients, who had lived in the area their entire lives, had a distinctive tooth stain known locally as "Colorado stain. [17] With the assistance of a dental researcher *G.V.Black*, it was found that histologically the enamel was imperfectly calcified and the affected teeth were less susceptible to dental caries than normal teeth [18].They implicated the water supplies is the etiology of the staining and pits. This staining is now known as dental fluorosis. After that, in 1933 a local dentist in Bauxite, USA noticed that children had mottled teeth. Thus, Mr. *H.V. Churchil* analyzed the water and found that the F ion concentration in the water supply of the Bauxite community was 13.7ppm, which is considered abnormally high [17].

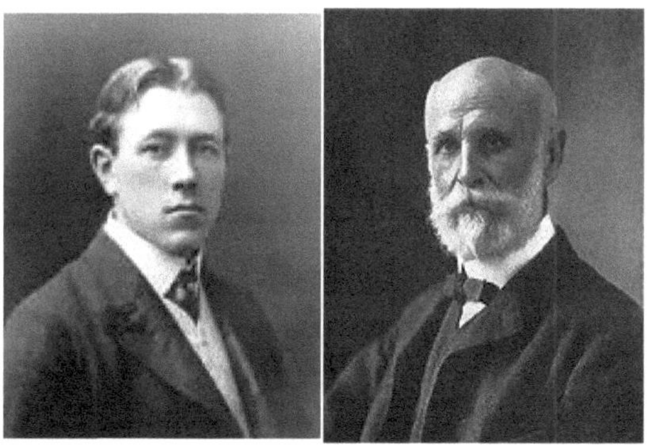

A B

Fig 2: A) Frederick McKay B) G.V. Black (Source: internet)

In 1938 extensive surveys of all communities affected by mottling in the USA conducted by *Dr Trendly Dean.* He found that when fluoride ion concentration was below 1 ppm, tooth mottling was either absent or minimal. Further studies in the USA indicated that at a fluoride concentration of 1 ppm, there was a reduction in dental caries without any associated tooth mottling. In 1944, Dean and his colleagues began testing the safety of artificially fluoridating water at this concentration. Finally, in 1953, it was reported that after six years of fluoridating the water in Grand Rapids, USA, dental caries was reduced by half compared to a control group. Since *Dr. Trendly Dean* discovered fluoride's anti-caries effect in 1938, fluoride has significantly contributed to the decline in the prevalence of dental caries. (18)

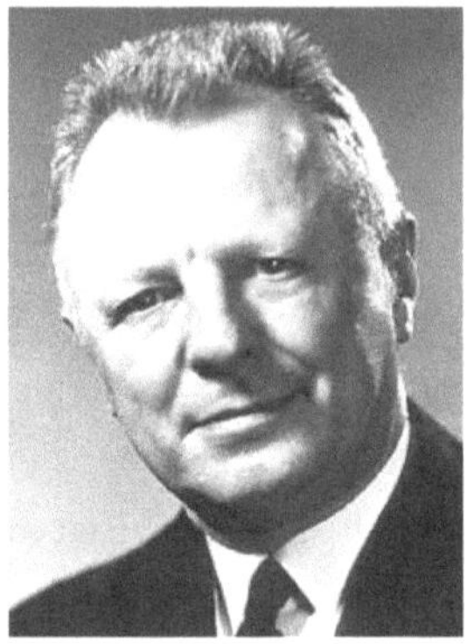

Fig 3: Dr Henry Trendly Dean (Source: internet)

1500s- Fluorine in the form of the calcium fluoride mineral fluorite was first mentioned in writings where it was used in metallurgy to assist working molten metals.

1901- McKay discovered the "Colorado stain". He named it "Mottled enamel".

1916- McKay and Black identified a community in Colorado Springs that had mottled enamel but unusually the teeth also showed a resistance to dental caries.

1916- Micro-abrasion first evolved from a technique previously carried out by Walker Kane but first described by Mc'Closkey and modified by Croll and Cavanaugh.

1930- McKay also showed in his 1930 study, that reports of mottled enamel similar to those that he and Dean had investigated, were being reported in many other parts of the world; South America, Mexico and North Africa were all cited which are all places known today to have water supplies affected with high levels of fluoride. McKay's 1930 paper also identified that the majority of the water sources identified with high levels of fluoride in the USA were from shallow or deep wells.

1930s- Fluorosis was first noticed in early 1930s, among cattle's by the farmers of Andhra Pradesh. They noticed inability of the bullocks to walk due to painful and stiff joints.

1931- The Science News journal published an article in which Dr. Margaret Cammack Smith claimed to have definitively proved the relationship between mottled teeth and fluoride in drinking water, speculating that poor nutrition could also exacerbate the condition.

1934- Trendley H Dean introduced the mottling index known as Dean's fluorosis index.

1937- Dean and Elvove said that could possibly be a level of fluoride in drinking water at which prevalence of caries could be reduced without the side of effect of dental fluorosis.

1937- The damaging effects of fluorine on bone from industrial exposure were observed in the 1930s (Roholm, 1937) by studying the effect of fluoride on bone, which later became known as skeletal fluorosis.

1938- A connection was identified linking drinking water with mottled enamel. This connection was demonstrated in a study published in 1938 which had monitored a community in Arkansas for 10 years following a change in the water supply, from a supply containing high fluoride to one containing a low level of fluoride (Dean and McKay, 1938).

1938- Dean and McKay showed that this action was successful in halting the occurrence of severe dental fluorosis.

1940s- Public health initiative of fluoridating public water supplies began.

1942- Dean et al discovered that at 1ppm F in drinking water, 60% reduction in dental caries was observed.

1944- (MacQuillian, 1944) In Tanzania, a study of chronic fluoride poisoning in the Arusha district was reported.

1946- A case study from China in 1946 identified bone deformities in a population drinking water high in fluoride, and although at this time it was not given the name skeletal fluorosis, it is clear from the descriptions that this was the case (Lyth, 1946).

1957- Dowse and Jenkins said that fluoride accumulates in early carious lesions.

1958- Zipkin et al found that fluoride of bone samples is more in tea drinking Britain than Americans.

1959- Smith and Hodge reported death after accidental ingestion of 2.5-5.0 g of Fluorides.

1959- Weidmann and Weatherall said that distribution of fluoride is more in the endosteum and periosteum.

1971- A study based in India describes endemic skeletal fluorosis and refers to a series of studies throughout the 1940s and 1950s (Teotia et al., 1971).

1971- Aasenden et al showed bouys have more fluoride uptake than girls.

1973- Moreno and Brudevold showed that contralateral teeth with the same exposure to Fluoride have similar concentrations and central incisors have lower fluoride concentration than laterals.

1974 - Barnhart said that the amount of fluoride ingested depends upon several factors, including the fluoride concentration of the product and may range from approximately 0.1 mg, in the case of dentifrices and mouth rinses, to more than 20 mg, in the case of professionally applied fluoride gels without proper suction

1976- Robinson and others were among the first to describe the infiltration technique for caries lesions using a resorcinol-formaldehyde resin.

1978- Thylstrup and Fejerskov index

1979- V. Ramasubramanian et al carried out a survey in seven states of India that were considered to have high levels of fluoride. It showed Andhra Pradesh and Gujarat had high levels of Fluoride.

1986- Croll and Cavanaugh described microabrasion.

1991- Belkir et al. suggested bleaching technique for fluorosis stain. Enamel is etched with 12% hydrochloric acid to remove the post-eruptive calcified surface enamel.

2004- Weinstein and Davison identified 8 main industrial sources which add to atmospheric fluoride. These are: aluminium smelting, petroleum refining, iron and steel production, phosphate fertilizer production, glass production and brick, ceramics and cement manufacture.

2009- Ozsvath described three main sources of fluoride in the environment; these are atmospheric, mineral and geothermal sources.

ETIOLOGY

There are multiple sources of fluoride and all have the potential to cause dental fluorosis – including natural fluoride, artificial or added fluoride in drinking water and dental products, as well as occupation- related exposures.

1) NATURAL SOURCES OF FLUORIDE CAUSING DENTAL FLUOROSIS

Dental fluorosis caused by high fluoride levels in underground water is a concern in certain regions of the world. In groundwater, fluoride can exist in an ionized form, and in areas with soil low in calcium, often found in regions rich in granite or gneiss elevated fluoride levels are typically observed. *Koparal et al* showed that human breast milk contains 0.019 +/- 0.004 ppm, while cow's milk has been shown to have fluoride levels of approximately 0.05 ppm. Other significant sources of fluoride include seafood and fruit juices. Tea leaves contain considerable amounts of fluoride and high consumption of tea is known to increase the risk of fluorosis. The bone of fish contains a large amount of fluoride and excessive consumption of fish with bone during tooth mineralization can cause fluorosis. Fruit juices, especially grape and orange juice, can be high in fluorides. [(19)]

In some areas, the atmosphere may contain high levels of fluoride from dust originating in fluoride-rich soils, as well as emissions from industries, underground coal fires, and volcanic activity. Estimates from 1992 suggested that about 1.4 million people in the United States had drinking water with natural fluoride concentrations between 2.0 and 3.9 mg/L, while just over 200,000 people had concentrations at or above the maximum contaminant level (MCL) of 4 mg/L. In 2000, it was estimated that approximately 162 million people had artificially fluoridated water (0.7-1.2 mg/L)[(19)]. Some areas have extremely high concentrations of fluoride in drinking water though water with levels higher that those recommended by the USEPA are monitored and are not used for human consumption. Alterations in physiological conditions; consumption of specific diets; disorder in acid–base balance; inhibition of carbonic anhydrase activity; iodine deficiency; poor nutritional status and usage of fluoride-rich food additives are identified as major predicting factors on the increased risk of dental fluorosis at high altitude regions[20]

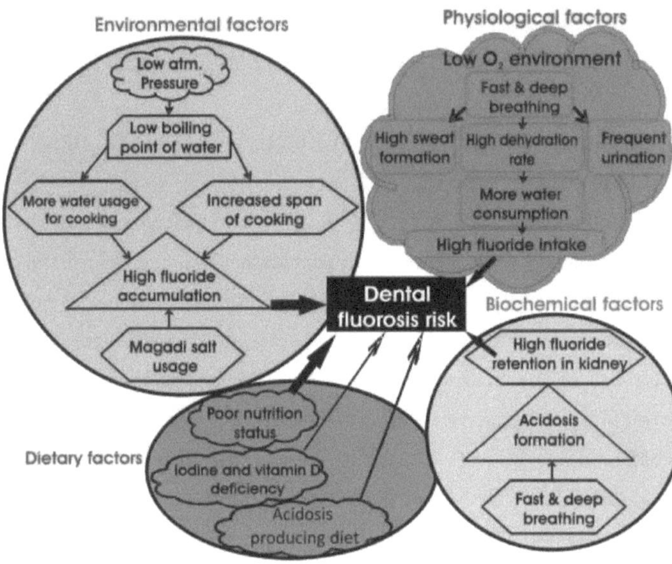

Fig 4: Factors causing fluorosis (source: Viswanathan G, Raja PB, Thirumoorthy K, Deepa R, Siva Ilango S. Pathways of factors exacerbating dental fluorosis risk at high altitude regions — A review. Environ Technol Innov. 2020

2) ADDITIONAL SOURCES OF FLUORIDE ASSOCIATED WITH DENTAL FLUOROSIS

Two primary sources have been identified as being potentially responsible for the prevalence of dental fluorosis:

- Fluoride in drinking water
- Fluoride containing dental products and supplements

A) FLUORIDE CONTAINING DRINKING WATER

Since 1945, fluoride has been used as a supplement in many public drinking water systems to help control dental decay. The US Centers for Disease Control and Prevention has recognized water fluoridation as one of the ten great public health achievements of the 20th century. However, with the increased use of fluoride in dental products (such as toothpaste, mouth rinses, and supplements) and its incorporation into food sources through fluoridated water, multiple sources of fluoride exposure have been linked to the rising incidence of dental fluorosis. Even a small 'pea- sized' amount of toothpaste containing 1,450 ppm fluoride, would contain approximately 0.36–0 .72 mg fluoride, which if consumed twice a day could contribute to fluoride levels that would increase the risk of dental fluorosis in children.(11)

Fluoridated water is directly or indirectly responsible for 40% of dental fluorosis, primarily through water consumption and the use of drinking water in infant formulas and food preparation. The remaining 60% of fluorosis cases are attributed to other fluoride sources. In a systematic review analyzing 214 studies, *Mc Donagh et al.* noted a reduction in the number of caries-affected teeth alongside an increase in dental fluorosis, which was related to varying levels of fluoride intake. They also stated that the prevalence of dental fluorosis indicates that children are ingesting other sources of fluoride besides drinking water.(21)

B) FLUORIDE CONTAINING DENTAL PRODUCTS AND SUPPLEMENTS

Fluoride supplements are recommended for children living in fluoride deficient areas. The recommended daily dose is based on children's age and on the concentration of fluoride in drinking water. Studies have identified fluoride supplements as a risk factor for dental fluorosis, both in fluoridated and non-fluoridated areas. In fluoridated areas, the risk of dental fluorosis from use of fluoride supplements is almost 4 times higher than in non-fluoridated areas. The risk of dental fluorosis originated from the use of fluoride supplements is well established.(3)

TOPICAL FLUORIDE

Types of topical Fluorides:

A) SELF-APPLIED

B) PROFESSIONALLY APPLIED

A) SELF-APPLIED FLUORIDE SUPPLEMENT

1. FLUORIDE TOOTHPASTE:

Fluoride-containing toothpaste is the most commonly used form of self-applied fluoride worldwide. Fluoride in toothpaste is absorbed directly by dental plaque and demineralized enamel, and it also elevates fluoride levels in saliva. Brushing with fluoride toothpaste can increase the fluoride concentration in saliva by 100 to 1,000 times. The active ingredient in fluoride-containing toothpastes can be sodium fluoride, sodium monofluorophosphate, or stannous fluoride. Fluoride toothpastes available over the counter generally contain a fluoride concentration of 1,000 to 1,500 ppm. Prescription-strength fluoride toothpastes contain 5,000 ppm fluoride as sodium fluoride.(3) *Naccache et al*, studied the variability in the ingestion of fluoride from toothpaste by preschool children, found that the amounts of toothpaste swallowed are widely variable and can be as much as 0.18 g to 0.33g.They also found that among children aged 12 to 24 months, 20% ingested more than 0.25 mg of fluoride per day by tooth brushing alone .Use of dentifrices flavored for children increases the quantity of toothpaste used and can increase the risk of swallowing the tooth paste . (3)

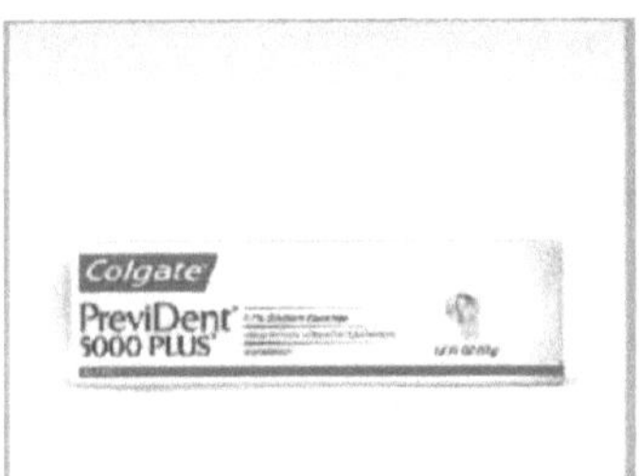

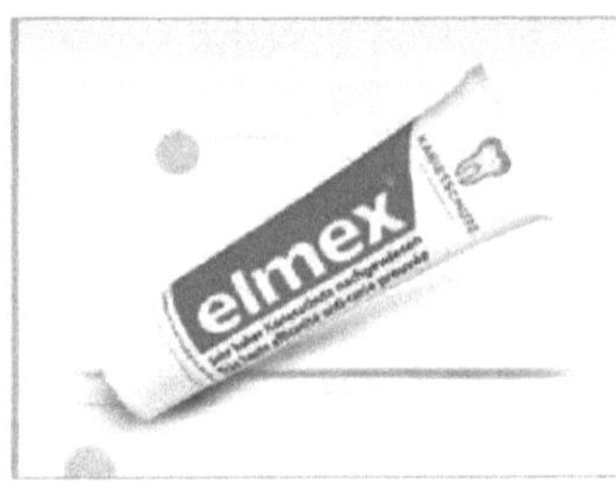

Fig 5: Fluoridated tooth pastes (Source: internet)

2. FLUORIDE MOUTHRINSE OR GELS:

Fluoride mouthrinse is a concentrated solution meant for daily or weekly use, designed to be rinsed and then spit out. The most commonly used fluoride compound in mouthrinse is sodium fluoride. Over-the-counter solutions containing 0.05% sodium fluoride (230 ppm fluoride) are available for individuals older than 6 years. Additionally, prescription options include self-applied gel formulations of sodium fluoride (1.1% or 5,000 ppm) and stannous fluoride (0.15% or 1,000 ppm) for home use. Studies have shown that 3-year olds swallow an average of 26 percent, 4-yearolds 24 percent, and 5 to 6 year olds 22 percent, each time they use mouth rinse. Currently, mouth rinses are not recommended for use by children under school age because of the risk of swallowing.(3)

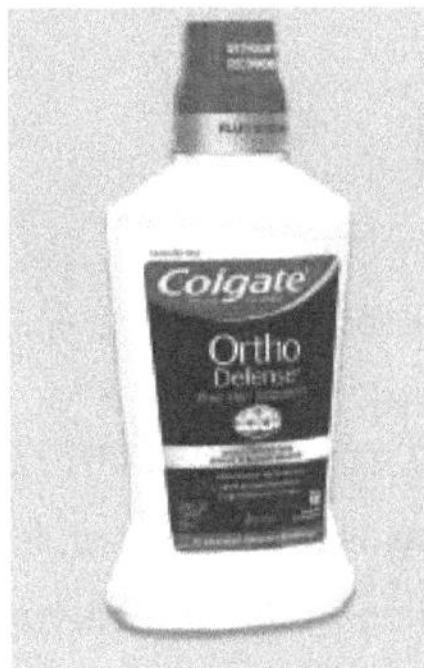

Fig 6: Fluoride mouthrinse pastes (Source: internet)

B) PROFESSIONALLY APPLIED FLUORIDE SUPPLEMENT

1. FLUORIDE GELS, OR FOAMS:

Professionally applied fluorides are in the form of a gel, foam or rinse, and are applied by a dental professional during dental visits. These fluorides are more concentrated than the self-applied fluorides (e.g., 1.23% fluoride ion [12,300 ppm]), and therefore are not needed as frequently. An early study reported that fluoride uptake by dental enamel increased in an acidic environment, fluoride gel is often formulated to be highly acidic (pH of approximately 3.0). Products available include gels of acidulated phosphate fluoride (1.23% [12,300 ppm] fluoride), as 2% neutral sodium fluoride products (containing 9,000 ppm fluoride), and as gels or foams of sodium fluoride (0.9% [9,040 ppm] fluoride). In a dental office, fluoride gel is generally applied for 1 to 4 minutes.(3)

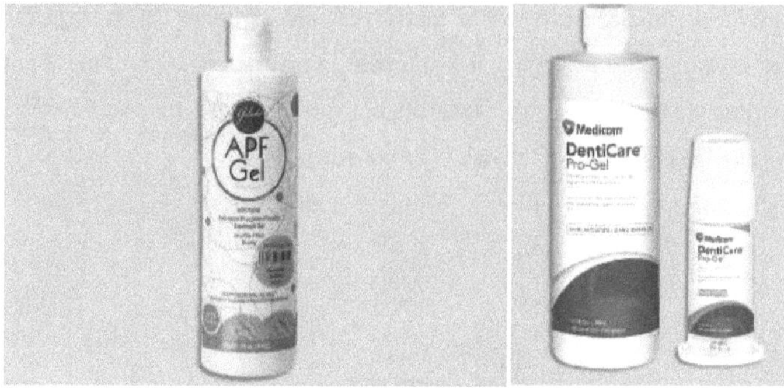

Fig 7: Fluoride Gels (Source: internet)

2. **FLUORIDE-CONTAINING PROPHYLAXIS PASTE**

Fluoride-containing paste is routinely used during dental prophylaxis. The abrasive paste, containing fluoride levels between 4,000 and 20,000 ppm, can help restore fluoride concentration in the enamel's surface layer that may have been lost during polishing. (3)

3. **FLUORIDE VARNISH**

Fluoride varnishes come in formulations such as sodium fluoride (2.26% or 22,600 ppm fluoride) and difluorsilane (0.1% or 1,000 ppm fluoride). A typical application involves 0.2 to 0.5 mL, delivering approximately 5 to 11 mg of fluoride ions.(3)

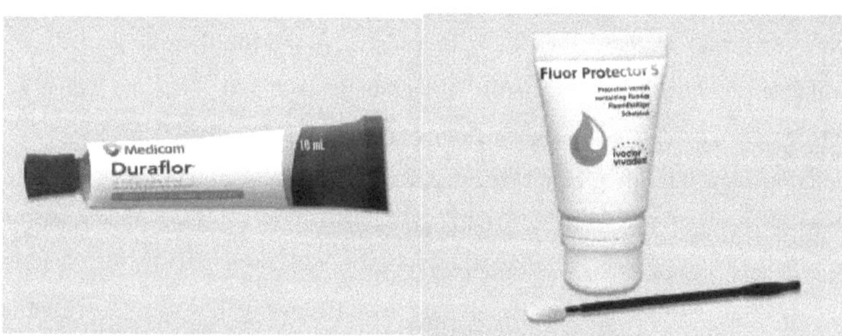

Fig 8: Fluoride Varnish (Source: internet)

4. **SILVER DIAMINE FLUORIDE**

Silver diamine fluoride (SDF) is a colorless liquid containing 24.4% to 28.8% silver (weight/volume) and 5.0% to 5.9% fluoride at a pH of 10. The FDA has classified SDF as a Class II medical device; it is cleared for use in the treatment of tooth sensitivity (which is the same type of clearance for fluoride varnish) and must be professionally applied. While some products are available in other countries, Advantage Arrest™ (Elevate Oral Care, L.L.C.) is currently the only commercially available silver diamine fluoride (SDF) product for dental use in the U.S.

Excessive fluoride intake, often due to improper use or swallowing of fluoride-containing toothpastes, contributes to the development of dental fluorosis. Children under 5 years old tend to swallow about 30% of the toothpaste used during brushing. When combined with the consumption of fluoridated water, this increases the potential risk of dental fluorosis The use of topical fluorides in young children is usually associated with inadvertent ingestion and systemic absorption of fluoride.[8] Although the very mild forms of dental fluorosis may not pose a public health problem, more severe forms will be of aesthetic concern, especially when the upper front teeth are involved. There is a need to get the appropriate balance between the beneficial and harmful effects of topical fluoride therapies.[22]

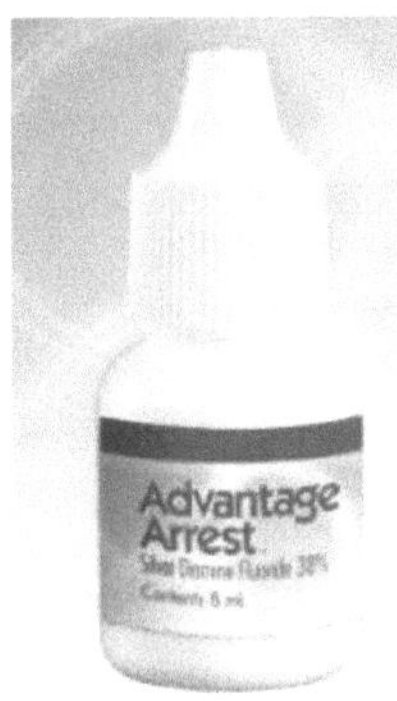

Fig 9: Silver diamine fluoride (SDF) (Source: internet)

C) OTHER FACTORS

1. EVIDENCE FOR GENETIC INFLUENCE ON FLUOROSIS

Currently, the literature on genetic determinants of dental fluorosis is limited. Some laboratory studies have demonstrated that the severity of dental fluorosis cannot be explained by the tooth concentration of fluoride. Some epidemiologic studies have found that prevalence of dental fluorosis was higher among African Americans than whites living in the same community, after adjusting for socioeconomic factors. [22]

Huang et al, in one of the few published studies that examined the influence of specific candidate genes, investigated the relationship between dental fluorosis and polymorphisms in the COL1A2 gene among children in china. They conducted a case-control study among children between 8 and 12 years of age with (n = 75) and without (n = 165) dental fluorosis. They found that the children who were homozygous for PP genotype of COL1A2 PvuII had a significantly increased risk of dental fluorosis when compared to children carrying the same genotype (pp) in an endemic fluorosis village.[22]

However, the risk was not elevated when the control population was recruited from a non-endemic fluorosis village. Their findings provide evidence of an association between polymorphisms in the COL1A2 gene with dental fluorosis in high fluoride exposed populations, which is evidence for presence of interaction between fluoride intake and the genotype. *Bretz et al* in their twin study in Brazil, found that there was a strong heritability component to dental fluorosis. In this study of 384 twin pairs, 95% of the variability of fluorosis occurrence was attributable to genetic factors.

It has also been demonstrated that fluoride affects the genes and gene pathways and proteins that play a role in development and mineralization of teeth. *Zhang et al* have shown that 10 µm sodium fluoride down-regulates expression of matrix metalloproteinase in human fetal tooth ameloblast-lineage cells, but did not alter the amount of amelogenin or 18allikrein-4 (KLK-4) synthesized by the cells. *Mousny et al,* investigated the genetic influence on bone susceptibility to fluoride. They studied three mice strains that demonstrate different susceptibilities to developing enamel fluorosis. These mice were divided into treatment groups receiving fluoride at concentrations of 0 ppm, 25 ppm, 50 ppm, 100 ppm. They found that fluoride treatment did not have much influence on BMD, but there were significant alterations in the quality of bone: there were significant alterations in "bone quality" in the A/J strain, moderate alterations in "bone quality" in the SWR/J strain and no effects in the 129P3/J strain. The results from their study suggest that genetic factors may contribute to the variation in bone response to fluoride intake and that fluoride might affect bone properties without altering BMD.[22]

2. MALNUTRITION

Massler et al, found that malnourished infants and children, especially if deficient in calcium intake, may have more severe forms of fluorosis than well-nourished children, even at the same levels of fluoride consumption. They suggested that, when an individual or a population group shows mottling beyond the degree expected, the health and nutritional status of that group should be investigated. *Yoder et al,* found the same relationship between malnutrition and severity of dental fluorosis in Tanzanian children.[23]

3. BEHAVIORAL FACTORS

Breastfeeding has been shown to have a protective effect against fluorosis. Feeding beyond 18 months of age has been shown to protect against dental fluorosis in permanent teeth. *Brothwell et al,* found that the prevalence of fluorosis was 27.2% in children breastfed for less than 6 months, 19.6% for those breastfed for 6-12 months, and 13.8% for those breastfed for more than 12 months. Additionally, disorders in acid-base balance can impact the kidneys' ability to manage fluoride. Thus, any factor that can decrease urinary pH would be expected to increase the likelihood of dental fluorosis and vice versa. Food products that change the pH of urine to alkaline can lead to increased excretion of fluoride and thereby decrease the risk of fluorosis. Food products that are rich in proteins are also known to have a protective effect against the effects of fluoride as they increase the excretion of fluoride from the body. Data from the Iowa Fluoride Study, indicated that amoxicillin could play a contributing role in the development of primary tooth fluorosis. In the case of the permanent dentition, they found a significant association between amoxicillin use during infancy and developmental enamel defects in the early-erupting permanent teeth after adjusting for fluoride intake and the length of breast feeding.[24]

MECHANISM OF ACTION OF FLUORIDE

From the 1940s to the 1970s, fluoride benefits were seen when this element was ingested from 'systemic' sources. Fluoride's action mostly depended on how it was absorbed by developing enamel. This would lead to the formation of fluorhydroxyapatite, a mineral phase more resistant to future dissolution Fluoride primarily affects the de- and re-mineralization processes occurring at the interface between the tooth surface and oral fluids through its topical impact. primary action of fluoride is topical due to its presence in the fluid phases of the oral environment.(6)

First, it can be useful to think about the various "pools" of fluoride that can be present in the oral environment. Five criteria can be used to didactically divide these pools.(25)

1) FO: outer fluoride, present outside enamel (in the biofilm or saliva);
2) FS: fluoride present in the solid phase, incorporated in the structure of the crystals, also known as fluorhydroxyapatite
3) FL: fluoride present at the enamel fluid;
4) FA: fluoride adsorbed to the crystal surface, also known as loosely- bound;
5) CaF_2: 'CaF_2- like' material; globules deposited on enamel and biofilm after application of highly concentrated fluoride products; acts as a pH controlled fluoride and calcium reservoir

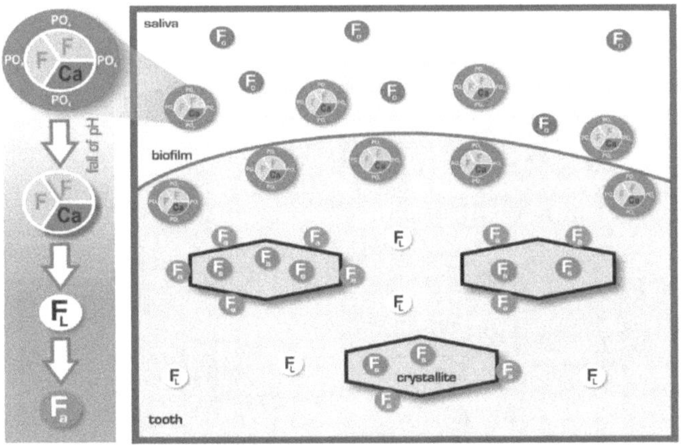

Fig 10: Schematic representation of the different 'pools' of fluoride in the oral environment. Modified from Arends and Christoffersen. (source: Arends J, Christoffersen J. Nature and role of loosely bound fluoride in dental caries. J Dent Res. 1990 Feb;69 Spec No:601–5; discussion 634-636.)

1) INHIBITION OF DEMINERALIZATION

If fluoride is present in plaque fluid (FL) when bacteria produce acids, it will penetrate along with the acids at the subsurface, adsorb to the crystal surface (FA) and protect crystals from dissolution. The higher the concentration of fluoride, the greater the likelihood of adsorption (FA), which helps protect the crystals. [26] Calcium fluoride (CaF_2) is an important source of fluoride to the oral fluids (FL). It is known as pH- controlled fluoride and calcium reservoir. This compound forms when the fluoride concentrations in the solution bathing enamel are higher than 100 ppm. The dissolution rate of CaF_2 globules is limited by the adsorption of HPO_4^{-2} that is lost under acidic pH, thus allowing CaF_2 to dissolve and fluoride and calcium to be released.[27] [28]

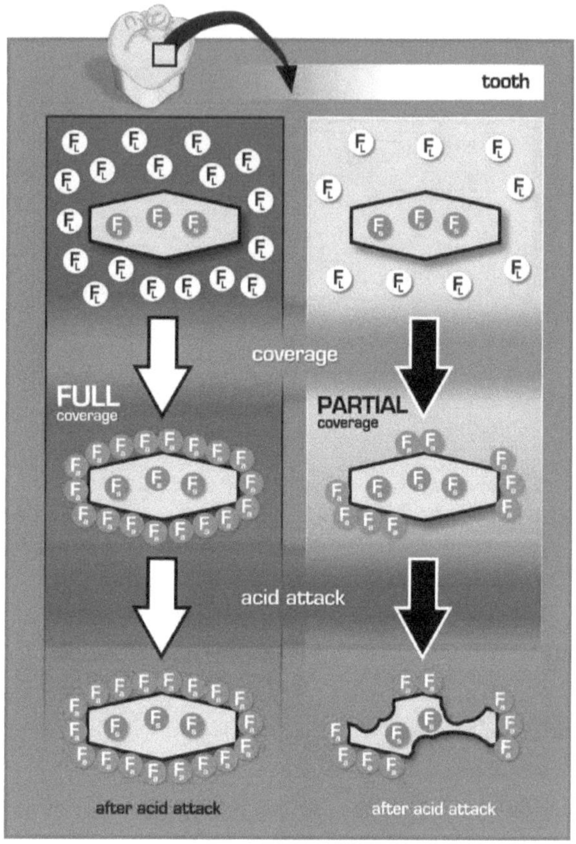

Fig 11: Events taking place at the subsurface of enamel upon a cariogenic acidic challenge. Fluoride (FL) penetrates at the subsurface along with the acids, adsorbs to the surface of the crystal and protects it from dissolution (left chart). When coverage is partial, uncovered portions of the crystal will dissolve (right chart). Modified from Arends and Christoffersen. (source: Arends J, Christoffersen J. Nature and role of loosely bound fluoride in dental caries. J Dent Res. 1990 Feb;69 Spec No:601–5; discussion 634-636.)

2) ENHANCEMENT OF REMINERALIZATION

Remineralization occurs naturally when the pH exceeds 5.5, as saliva is rich in tooth minerals. Additionally, if fluoride is present during the dissolution of hydroxyapatite, the solution will become highly supersaturated with fluorhydroxyapatite. This will hasten the remineralization process. The partially demineralized crystals will bind fluoride to their surface and draw calcium ions. Since carbonate-free or low-carbonate apatite is less soluble, these phases are more likely to develop under the nucleating action of partially dissolved minerals than the original mineral. Due to the inclusion of fluoride and the inclusion of carbonate, this new coating will be less soluble, making the enamel more resistant to future acidic challenges. The effectiveness of water fluoridation in controlling tooth decay can be attributed to the frequent contact of fluoride with the tooth structure or intraoral fluoride reservoirs. Since fluoridated water is consumed multiple times a day, this high frequency of contact helps explains why even though the fluoride concentrations in water are much lower than those in fluoride toothpastes, for example, water fluoridation remains highly effective in caries control. This principle can be applied to all systemic methods of fluoride use.[28] [26]

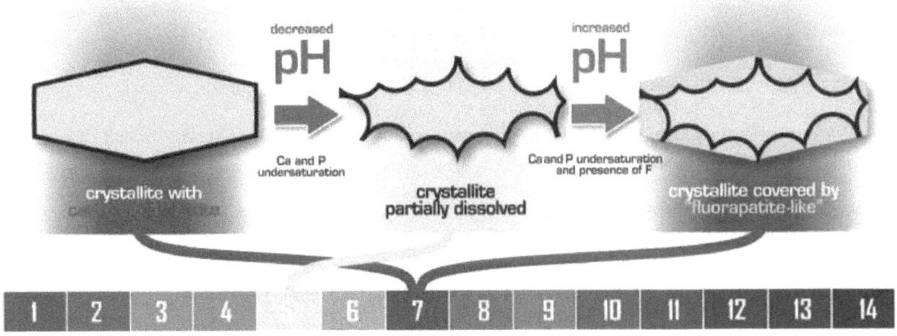

Fig 12: Schematic representation of remineralization occurring in the presence of fluoride. Fluoride speeds up the process of remineralization and leads to the precipitation of a coat poor in carbonate and rich in fluoride on the partially demineralized original crystallite. This renders the tooth structure more resistant to subsequent acidic challenges. (source: Arends J, Christoffersen J. Nature and role of loosely bound fluoride in dental caries. J Dent Res. 1990 Feb;69 Spec No:601–5; discussion 634-636.)

3) EFFECTS IN ORAL BACTERIA

The physiology of microbial cells, particularly cariogenic streptococci, can be impacted by fluoride ions, which may consequently indirectly affect demineralization. By directly inhibiting cellular enzymes (either alone or in conjunction with metals), fluoride has an impact on oral bacteria. It also increases the proton permeability of cell membranes in the form of hydrogen fluoride (HF), which has an impact on bacteria. Glycolysis produces less acid as a result of intracellular F-'s inhibition of glycolytic enzymes. Acid generation and acid tolerance in S. mutans are both impacted by F- in the cytoplasm, which likewise reduces cytoplasmic pH. [29]

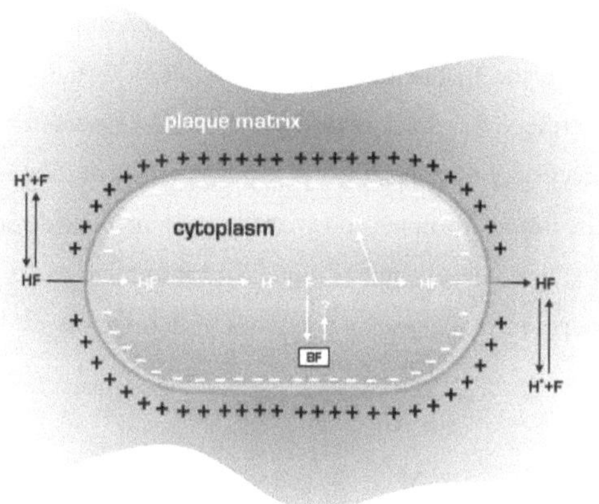

Fig 13: Fluoride accumulation, distribution and efflux from bacterial cells. BF=Bound fluoride. (source: Arends J, Christoffersen J. Nature and role of loosely bound fluoride in dental caries. J Dent Res. 1990 Feb;69 Spec No:601–5; discussion 634-636.)

BIOLOGICAL EFFECTS AND MECHANISMS OF ACTION OF FLUORIDE ON ORAL BACTERIA

Biological activity	Examples	Mechanism
Enzyme inhibition (at sub-millimolar levels of fluoride)	enolase, urease, P-ATPase, phosphatases, heme catalase, heme peroxidase	direct binding of F^- or HF
	F-ATPase, nitrogenase, RecA, CheY	binding of metal-F complex
Dissipation of proton gradient/ motive force (at micromolar levels of fluoride)	acidification of cytoplasm (inhibition of glycolysis, PTS system, and IPS formation)	action as transmembrane proton carrier
	inhibition of macromolecular synthesis and export	

PTS system = Phosphotransferase sugar transport system; IPS formation = intracellular polysaccharide formation. Source: Koo [33].

Table 1: (source: Arends J, Christoffersen J. Nature and role of loosely bound fluoride in dental caries. J Dent Res. 1990 Feb;69 Spec No:6 01–5; discussion 634-636.)

4) INCREASED ENAMEL RESISTANCE /REDUCED ENAMEL SOLUBILITY

There are three principle forms of fluoride ion reactivity with apatite:

1) Iso-ionic exchange of F- for OH- in apatite:

$$Ca_{10}(PO_4)_6(OH)_2 + 2F^- \rightarrow Ca_{10}(PO_4)_6F_2 + 2OH^-$$

2) Crystal growth of fluorapatite from supersaturated solutions:

$$10\ Ca^{2+} + 6PO_4^{\ 3-} + 2F^- \rightarrow Ca_{10}(PO_4)_6F_2$$

3) Apatite dissolution with CaF_2 formation:

$$Ca_{10}(PO_4)_6(OH)_2 + 20F^- \rightarrow 10\ CaF_2 + 6PO_4^{\ 3-} + 2OH$$

These reactions result in fluoride incorporation that would be defined as "firmly" bound fluoride The solid phase's fluoride is also referred to as fluorhydroxyapatite. CaF_2 is produced as a reaction product at fluoride concentrations between 100 and 10,000 ppm F. After a topical fluoride application, calcium fluoride can remain on the surface of teeth for weeks or months because it is somewhat insoluble in saliva at neutral pH. At neutral pH, secondary phosphate (HPO_4^{2-}) adsorption to calcium sites on the surface of calcium fluoride crystals and pellicle proteins are thought to be the causes of calcium fluoride's resistance. Fluoride ions released during cariogenic challenges are a result of the decreased concentration of secondary phosphate ions at acid pH. Consequently, calcium fluoride serves as a pH-controlled reservoir of fluoride on the enamel.[(6)]

DISTRIBUTION OF FLUORIDE IN ORAL CAVITY

Fluoride exposure leads to a slightly elevated steady-state level of fluoride in oral fluids, primarily found in saliva and plaque fluid. Fluoride can exist in various forms and compartments within the oral cavity. It may be ionized in saliva, ionized in plaque (plaque fluid), bound in plaque, bound as calcium fluoride, bound to enamel, and bound to soft tissues. Through diffusion, fluoride is distributed to oral tissues and dental plaque.[30]

After fluoride exposure, plaque acts as a reservoir, storing and releasing fluoride over time. The concentration of fluoride in saliva is typically around 0.6 mmol/L (0.01 ppm), although this value can vary depending on factors such as the use of fluoridated toothpaste, other fluoride-containing agents, and food items. [31] There can be significant diurnal variation in salivary fluoride concentration. For children living in areas with a water supply containing 1.2 ppm fluoride.

The fluoride concentration in saliva is independent of salivary flow rate. In unstimulated and stimulated parotid saliva, submandibular/sublingual saliva, and whole saliva, the fluoride concentration is approximately two-thirds of the simultaneously collected plasma fluoride concentration. The salivary fluoride concentration has been observed to range between 0.5 and roughly 2.0 mmol/L throughout the day.[32] This relationship remains consistent even when the plasma fluoride concentration is increased due to fluoride ingestion. [31]

Overall, fluoride distribution in the oral cavity is complex, with saliva and plaque playing crucial roles in the storage and release of fluoride. The concentration of fluoride in saliva can vary depending on multiple factors, and the relationship between saliva and plasma fluoride concentrations is maintained across different salivary glands and saliva types. The fluoride concentration in plaque can vary from 1 to about 10 ppm.[33] In plaque fluid, the baseline level of fluoride typically ranges from 15 to 17 mmol/L, which is approximately 30 times higher than the baseline value found in saliva.[34] The distribution and clearance of fluoride from various sites within the oral cavity are connected to the access of saliva to these sites. These site-specific differences in fluoride distribution may have clinical implications, particularly in relation to the dynamics of demineralization and remineralization processes.[35]

Plaque acts as a reservoir for fluoride storage and release, and the higher fluoride concentrations in plaque fluid compared to saliva indicate its potential impact on the surrounding oral tissues. The distribution of fluoride within plaque and its interaction with saliva can influence the availability of fluoride for protecting tooth surfaces against demineralization (tooth decay) and promoting remineralization (repair of early tooth decay). The clearance and distribution of fluoride in the oral cavity, influenced by salivary access to different sites, can impact the efficacy of fluoride in preventing tooth decay and supporting tooth remineralization. The clinical consequences of these site-specific differences in fluoride dynamics can help shape preventive strategies and treatment approaches to maintain optimal oral health. The distribution and clearance of fluoride in the oral cavity, including variations in plaque and saliva fluoride concentrations, are linked to salivary access to different sites. These site-specific differences may have clinical implications for the dynamics of fluoride in the processes of demineralization and remineralization, and understanding these dynamics can guide preventive and treatment strategies for maintaining oral health. [30]

Fluoride is rapidly and extensively absorbed from the gastrointestinal tract after ingestion. From the bloodstream, fluoride is removed through uptake by calcified tissues (such as teeth and bones) and excretion through the urine. Approximately 99% of the body's fluoride burden is associated with calcified tissues, and most of it is not easily exchangeable. Dentin and bone tend to have similar fluoride concentrations, which increase with age, while enamel has significantly lower fluoride levels.[36] Surface enamel fluoride concentrations typically decrease with age in areas of tooth wear, but they increase in areas that accumulate plaque. Dentin fluoride levels gradually decline from the pulpal surface towards the dentin-enamel junction (DEJ). Enamel fluoride concentrations are highest at the surface and progressively decrease towards the DEJ. Bulk enamel fluoride concentrations mainly reflect the level of fluoride exposure during tooth formation, while dentin and bone fluoride concentrations generally reflect the long-term intake of fluoride. [37]

These findings indicate that the distribution and concentration of fluoride in different dental tissues vary. Enamel, dentin, and bone all play important roles in fluoride storage and retention. The patterns of fluoride concentration in dental tissues can provide insights into the individual's fluoride exposure history and the potential impact on tooth health and development.(36) In general, the concentration of fluoride (F) in dental tissues follows certain patterns. An elevated concentration of fluoride is typically found at the anatomical surfaces of all three dental tissues (enamel, dentin, and cementum), while interior concentrations are generally lower. However, in cementum, there is often a smooth transition across the cementum-dentin junction (CDJ), with a negative gradient from surface to interior that disregards the histological boundary. (38) At the enamel-dentin junction (EDJ), the pattern is different. Previous reports indicate that fluoride concentrations tend to rise slightly from the interior of the enamel towards the EDJ, and in some cases, a similar tendency is observed on the dentinal side of this junction. These small peaks could be related to a zone of hypermineralization formed at the EDJ during development or indicate a tendency for the EDJ to leak, allowing fluoride and other substances to diffuse along it, similar to the way caries spreads along the EDJ.(39)

In dentin and cementum, the average fluoride content increases with age. It is unclear whether this increase is primarily due to higher concentrations at the surface or an overall increase throughout the tissue, as this study had a limited number of teeth.(38) Cementum has a higher fluoride concentration compared to other skeletal or dental tissues, which may be attributed to its thin structure adjacent to a large anatomical surface, making it readily accessible to fluoride.(40) The total fluoride content in dentin and cementum, which also increases with age, partially reflects their increasing thickness. There were no indications of age-related changes in the fluoride content of enamel. In enamel, the fluoride concentration is consistently highest in the outermost region. Typically, there is an exponential decrease in concentration towards a plateau in the inner third of the enamel. Then, the fluoride concentration slightly increases again across the final 50 micrometers or so towards the EDJ. In coronal dentin, fluoride concentrations throughout the tissue are higher than in enamel. At approximately 300 micrometers from the pulp cavity, there is a significant increase in fluoride concentration towards the pulpal surface.

In cementum, fluoride concentrations are highest at or near the surface of the root and decrease towards the interior.[38] Gingival crevicular fluid (GCF) tends to have slightly higher fluoride levels compared to plasma. On the other hand, concentrations in parotid and submandibular ductal saliva show a slight decrease, with ratios of ductal saliva and plasma fluoride concentrations around 0.8-0.9. This indicates that GCF may have a greater fluoride concentration compared to saliva. Whole saliva, however, often exhibits more variability and higher fluoride levels compared to ductal saliva due to contamination from external sources such as food, water, and fluoridated dental products. [36]

In the tooth structure, higher fluoride concentrations are found in the pulp, which gradually decreases as it approaches the dentin-enamel junction (DEJ).[41] Enamel fluoride content also increases with age, but it is comparatively lower and unrelated to dentin fluoride levels.[42] Generally, the fluoride concentration in tooth enamel reflects fluoride exposure during the process of amelogenesis.[41] However, while enamel is the target tissue for dental fluorosis, there is no established correlation between fluoride content in enamel and the occurrence of fluorosis. [42]

PATHOPHYSIOLOGY

In studying the pathophysiology of this widespread condition, we can conclude that it involves the interaction between fluorine and the outermost layer of tooth structure, known as enamel. This element is found naturally in nature, in water, in soil, and in many foods as well. This element has previously shown that it has led to prevention of caries by making the outermost layer strong enough and also by making the outermost layer super resistant to the attacks in oral cavity by acids and several other attacks. A more than normal quantity of exposure can further lead to dental fluorosis.(43) (44)While the stages of tooth development procedures are ongoing, formation of enamel occurs and this enamel contains crystals of hydroxyapatite which are deposited on the outermost layer. Fluoride can disrupt this process by interfering with crystal formation, ultimately resulting in an abnormal structure of the enamel. The proper mechanism is much more complicated than the normal mechanism which is described here but it is said that the enzymes which hampers the formation of these crystals along with the mineralization are somewhere interrupted by this element.(11)

The severity of dental fluorosis in a tooth is influenced by the amount of fluoride consumed, the duration of exposure, and the time since that exposure occurred. Mild dental fluorosis may manifest as white spots or streaks on the surface of the tooth. Severe fluorosis in the other hand can lead to excessive discoloration and excessive pitting on the surface of enamel.(45)

NORMAL ENAMEL DEVELOPMENT

It is necessary to understand the mechanisms controlling normal enamel formation to determine how fluoride affects enamel development. Dental enamel is formed by the ameloblasts, which are cells that differentiate from the dental lamina. The ameloblasts differentiate into polarized cells and begin to secrete an extracellular matrix. The morphologic features of the ameloblasts and the appearance of the extracellular matrix which they produce have been used to define the stages of enamel development. Although various classifications for stages of enamel formation exist, the stages are most often identified as pre-secretory,

secretory, transition, and maturation. During the pre-secretory stage, the differentiating ameloblasts acquire their phenotype and prepare to secrete the organic matrix of enamel. In the secretory stage, the secreted protein consists primarily of amelogenins, which are hydrophobic proteins that are later removed from the maturing enamel matrix. Other proteins, such as tuftelin, enamelin, ameloblastins, and metalloproteinases, are secreted. in lesser quantities. As the secretory stage continues, these matrix proteins begin to be hydrolyzed. The cells then shorten into transition-stage ameloblasts and begin to secrete proteinases, which begin a rapid degradation of amelogenins. The early-maturation stage follows, with a highly porous matrix overlaid with maturation stage ameloblasts. The maturation stage is characterized by modulating cycles of ruffle-bordered and smooth-bordered ameloblasts. These cells remove the rest of the amelogenin from the maturing enamel matrix and direct the final mineralization of the enamel. At the end of maturation, the cells lose their polarity and become the reduced enamel epithelium, which is lost from the surface of the tooth when the tooth erupts into the oral cavity. (11)

STAGES OF TOOTH FORMATION AND STAGE-SPECIFIC EFFECTS OF CHRONIC FLUORIDE EXPOSURE

pre-secretory ameloblasts differentiate into secretory ameloblasts after the dentin matrix begins to mineralize. The pre-secretory ameloblasts and surrounding enamel cells, including the enamel knot, are believed to play a role in tooth morphogenesis. (46) However, studies have shown no evidence that exposure to physiological levels of fluoride in vivo and in organ culture affects tooth morphogenesis. Even in teeth with severe fluorosis, the size and form of the teeth are not changed (47)

As pre-ameloblasts differentiate into secretory ameloblasts, they begin to secrete enamel matrix proteins, creating a thin layer of aprismatic enamel against the mantle dentin. Once the secretory ameloblasts' Tomes' processes develop, the inner enamel layer, which makes up the majority of the enamel, begins to form. This enamel matrix consists of prismatic enamel, with both rod (or prism) and inter-rod structures (inter-prismatic enamel) produced by the fully differentiated secretory ameloblasts. These cells secrete matrix protein (predominantly amelogenins) into the enamel space through which thin but long enamel crystals grow preferentially in length in the wake of the retreating cells.[11] Secretory stage ameloblasts exposed to high chronic levels of fluoride have a somewhat disrupted morphology and increased numbers of vacuoles at the apical border. Chronic exposure to fluoride in drinking water or repeated injections of moderate fluoride doses reduces the thickness of enamel by about 10% .the small reduction in enamel thickness may be attributed to a limited disruption of vesicular transport in fluorotic secretory ameloblasts and subsequent intracellular degradation of a minor portion of the matrix by the lysosomal system .[48]

At the conclusion of enamel secretion, ameloblasts lose their Tomes' processes and deposit a final layer of aprismatic enamel containing small crystals. During a brief transitional phase, the enamel matrix proteins are rapidly broken down, resulting in the porous enamel matrix typical of this stage. Notably, the late secretory-transitional stage ameloblasts seem to be more sensitive to fluoride compared to early and fully secretory ameloblasts. In hamster molar tooth germs, a dose of 4.5 mg/kg fluoride induces the late secretory to transitional cells, but not early secretory ameloblasts to detach occasionally from the surface and form sub-ameloblastic cysts. The enamel below the cysts under late secretory ameloblasts will give rise to the shallow occlusal pits, often seen in severely fluorosed teeth in various species.[47] This stage of development is likely also to be associated with the formation of accentuated perikymata that is clinically the first sign of enamel fluorosis. In the maturation stage, the ameloblasts modulate cyclically from cells with a smooth-ended to a ruffle ended distal membrane, the latter with characteristics of resorbing cells. During this modulation, matrix proteins continue to be removed from the extracellular space, and mineralization increases to form a fully mineralized enamel matrix. Amelogenin proteins are retained in the fluorosed rat enamel matrix at this stage of enamel formation [49], [50].

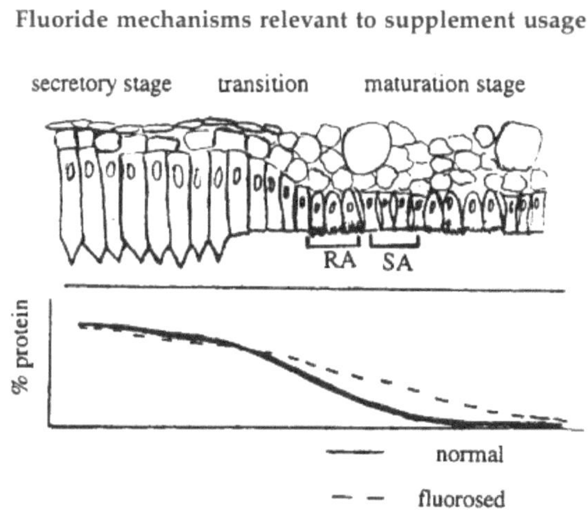

Fig 14: Diagram of ameloblasts showing the cell morphology at different developmental stages. The relative amount of protein in the enamel matrix corresponding to the ameloblast morphology, is shown in the graph below. The protein content of fluorosed enamel is higher at the transition and early maturation stages of formation, as compared to normal enamel. RA, ruffle-ended ameloblasts; SA, smooth-ended ameloblasts. (source: DenBesten PK: Biological mechanisms of dental fluorosis relevant to the use of fluoride supplements. Community Dent Oral Epidemiol 1999; 27: 41–7.)

EFFECTS OF FLUORIDE ON ENAMEL DEVELOPMENT

1. EFFECTS ON CELL FUNCTION

At high levels of fluoride, a major effect appears to be the reduced secretion of enamel proteins.[(51) (49) (52)] However, this effect of fluoride on secretory stage enamel appears to be mostly reversible. The primary effects of fluoride occur during the early maturation stage, when fluoride can rapidly accumulate. [(52)] Chronic exposure of animals to high levels of fluoride in their food or water causes multiple effects on amelogenesis, including the induction of abnormal modulation cycles within maturation stage ameloblasts. The number of cycles decreases in a dose-dependent manner with increasing levels of fluoride exposure. [(53) (46)] .Alterations in the modulation of ameloblasts would affect the processing of the matrix proteins and subsequent mineralization of the mature enamel.

2. EFFECTS ON MATRIX MINERALIZATION

The beginning of enamel maturation is defined by a secondary influx of mineral ions and is characterized by a white opaque zone which was described in rat incisors by *Hiller et al.* [54] and later shown to be present in most species . The white opaque zone and the preceding transitional enamel are also characterized by a selective uptake of fluoride [55], possibly because of the high degree of hydration at this stage which would allow free access to the tissue . The increased uptake of fluoride at this stage may partly explain the susceptibility of early-maturation enamel to the effects of fluoride. The relatively high concentrations of fluoride that are found in the enamel matrix at the transition/early-maturation stage of enamel formation could reduce the availability of ionic calcium, resulting in reduced proteolytic activity at this critical stage .[56]

A study by Bronckers and co-workers [51] of the effects of fluoride on the mineralization of hamster molars in tooth organ culture showed that fluoride in the medium irreversibly affected the existing mineralizing matrix by producing a rapid deposition of crystals and disrupting their growth. Furthermore, fluoride in the medium interfered with the deposition of crystals in the new matrix. However, when fluoride was removed from the medium, the newly formed matrix recovered and mineralized normally. These findings suggest that fluoride may interfere with the nucleating sites.[57] After exposure to fluoride, the nature of the mineral component of enamel is altered. Fluorosed enamel has an increased concentration of magnesium and in bone mineral, fluoride increases manganese and decreases concentrations of carbonate, citrate [37], and zinc. These changes in the mineral chemistry could affect mineral-matrix interactions and enzyme activity. For example, it has been suggested that enamel proteins produced in the presence of fluoride may be more tightly bound to fluoroapatite, thereby making them less accessible to degradation by enamel proteinases.[58]

The mechanism responsible for the delay in hydrolysis and removal of amelogenin has not yet been determined. However, fluoride may alter the quantity or activity of extracellular proteinases needed to degrade enamel proteins during the maturation stage of amelogenesis. Although proteinases are present in the enamel in both the secretory and the maturation stages, the proteinases most active in the hydrolysis of amelogenin are the serine proteinases, which are present at the maturation stage. There is some evidence to suggest that the proteolytic activity of serine proteinases is reduced in fluorosed enamel, compared to normal enamel. The delayed removal of amelogenin may be an important mechanism in the development of fluorosis by delaying the growth of enamel crystals, so that when the tooth erupts, the enamel remains incompletely mineralized.(59,60)

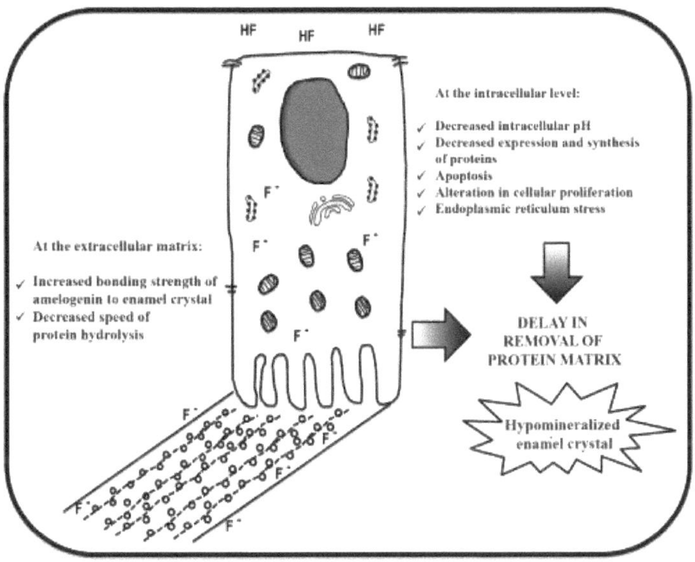

Fig 15: Possible biochemical and cellular mechanisms involved in the pathogenesis of dental fluorosis, both at the intracellular level and the extracellular matrix (source: Castiblanco G. Pathogenesis of Dental Fluorosis: Biochemical And Cellular Mechanisms. Rev Fac Odontol Univ Antioquia. 2017 Jun 1; 28:408.)

HISTOPATHOLOGY

Histopathologically, non-pitted fluorotic enamel shows a subsurface porosity below a well-mineralized surface zone. This subsurface porosity is what produces the whiter, more opaque appearance of the enamel. With increasingly severe fluorosis, the porosity extends toward the dentinal enamel junction, and the enamel surface can break down after eruption, resulting in pitting of the enamel. *Fejerskov* and co-workers have shown that the severity of dental fluorosis is directly related to the amount of fluoride in the enamel, and the subsurface porosity.(61)

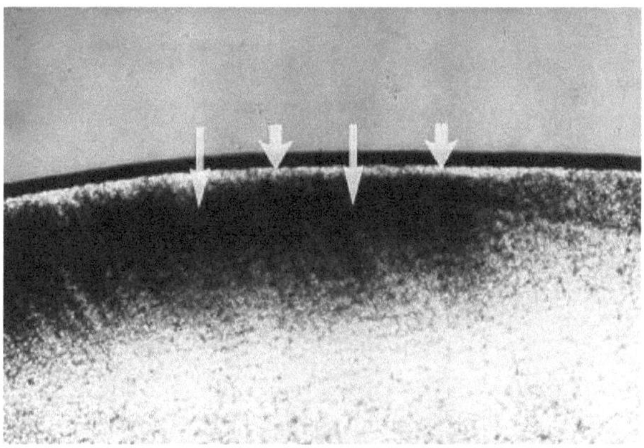

Fig 16: Polarized light micrograph of fluorosed enamel in water. The well-mineralized (negatively birefringent) surface layer is indicated by the shorter arrows, and the hypomineralized (positively birefringent) subsurface layer, characteristic of fluorosed enamel, is indicated by the longer arrows.(source: DenBesten PK: Biological mechanisms of dental fluorosis relevant to the use of fluoride supplements. Community Dent Oral Epidemiol 1999; 27: 41–7.)

I. ENAMEL

Figure 17 shows teeth with mild fluorosis; enamel showed thin areas which were white in the subsurface due to demineralization. In fluorosed teeth, the thickness of enamel was comparatively less and demineralization was seen as light-yellow and brown shade as shown.(61)

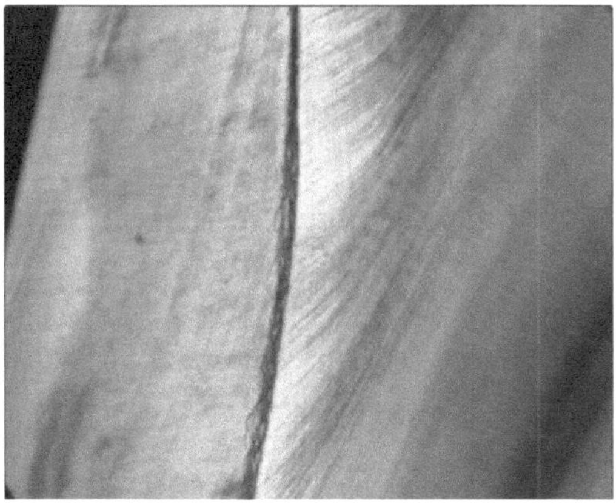

Fig: 17 Enamel showed thin areas which were white in the subsurface due to demineralization

In figure 18 fluorosis, mild demineralization was seen as light shade in the cuspal area of enamel with disturbance in gnarled enamel pattern.

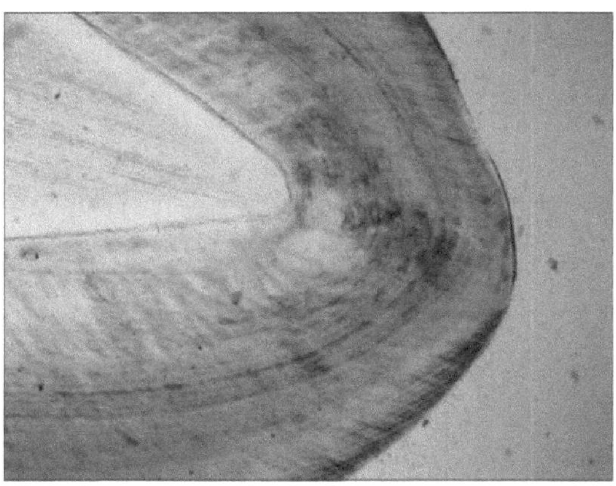

Fig 18: Mild de-mineralization in DEJ in cusp and disturbance in gnarled enamel pattern

In moderate and severe fluorosis, the whiter areas in enamel were broader representing more areas of demineralization and they were evident in the deeper areas of the enamel as shown in Figures 19 and 20.[61]

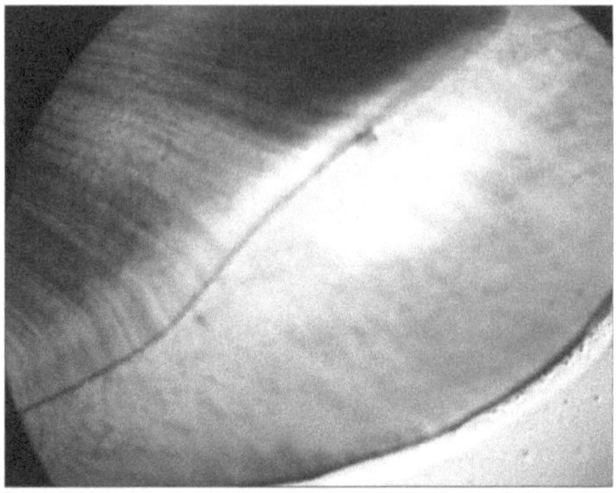

Fig 19: Moderate Dental fluorosis - whiter areas becoming broader representing more areas of demineralization in deeper areas

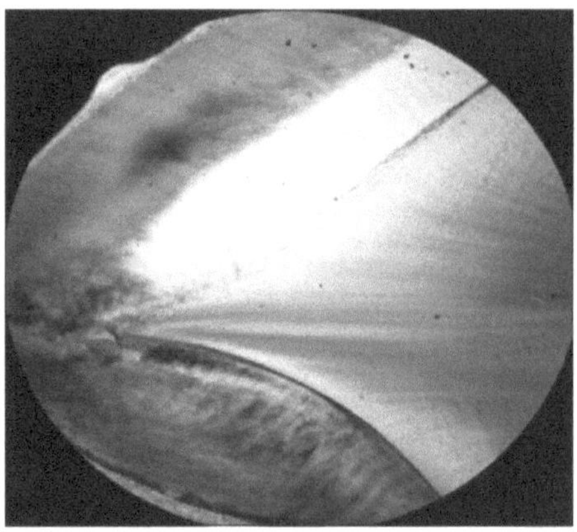

Fig 20: Moderate demineralization near dentinoenamel junction

In severe fluorosis, as seen in figure 21 dentinoenamel junction (DEJ) was not scalloped but irregular. Intermingling of crystals was seen in the junction between dentin and enamel.[61]

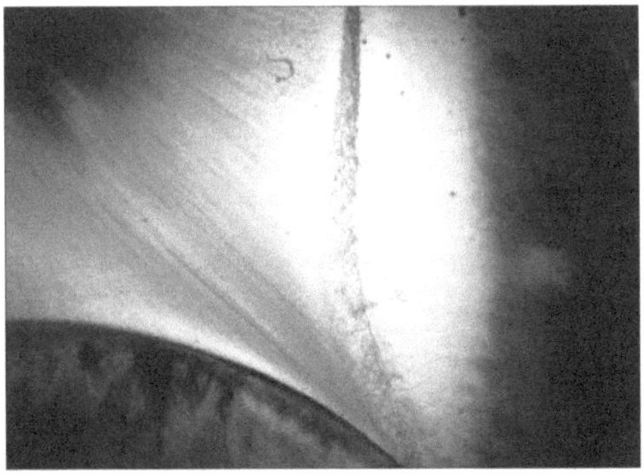

Fig 21 :Severe dental fluorosis

In sections of moderate and severe fluorosis, broadening of incremental lines was seen figure 22.

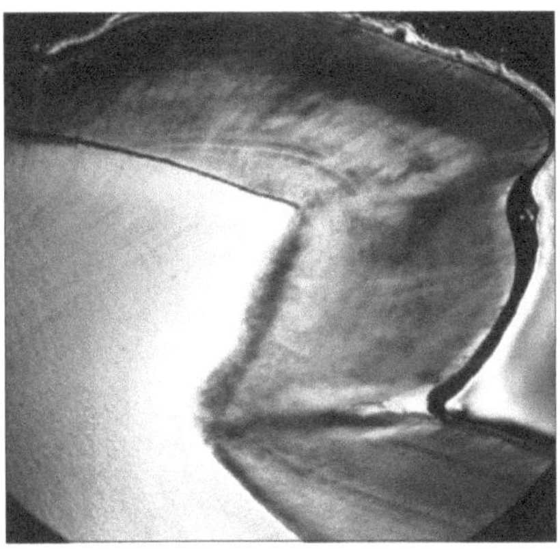

Fig 22: Moderate and Severe with darker and broader incremental lines

Figure 23 shows severe demineralization, and hole damage was seen in enamel with Grade 4 DF

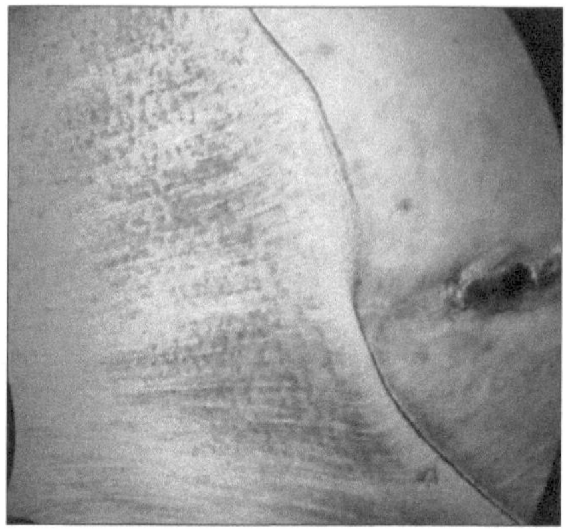

Fig 23: Severe dental fluorosis with hole damage seen in enamel

II. DENTIN

In Figure 24, dentinal tubules without fluorosis showed a gentle curve in the crown resembling "S" which is less in the root called as primary curvatures. [61]

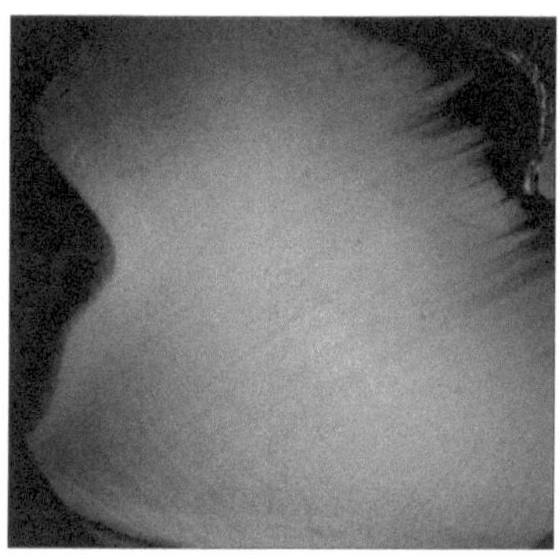

Fig 24: Normal dentinal tubules

The dentinal tubules were more irregular and curved in fluorosed teeth as shown in Figure 25

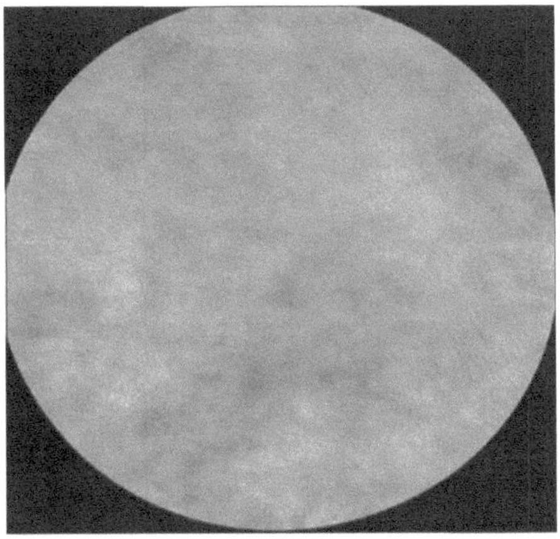

Fig 25: Irregular and curved dentinal tubules in Dental fluorosis

Some of the fluorosed teeth with higher grades showed more amount of inter-globular dentin as shown in Figure 26 with numerous dead tracts as shown in Figure 27

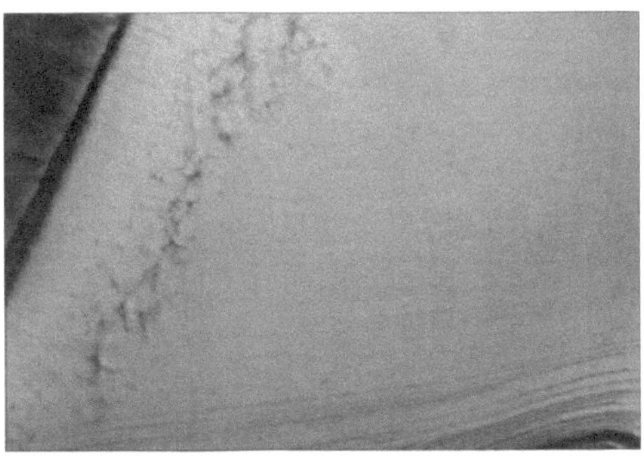

Fig 26 More interglobular dentin

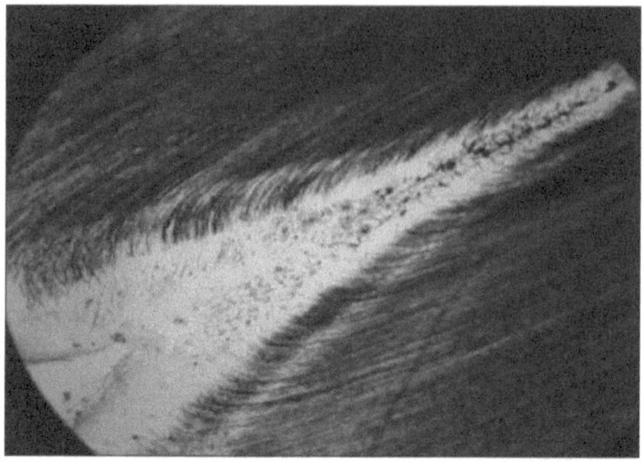

Fig 27 : Dental fluorosis with more dead tracts

Figure 28 shows secondary curvatures which were found to be numerous in fluorosed teeth.

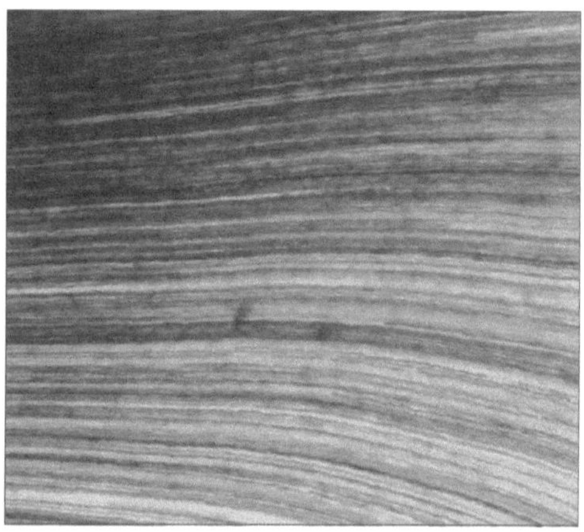

Fig 28: Dental fluorosis with numerous secondary curvatures

III. RADICULAR PORTION

The cementodentinal junction was diffuse and irregular in higher grades of fluorosis as shown in Figure 29 [61]

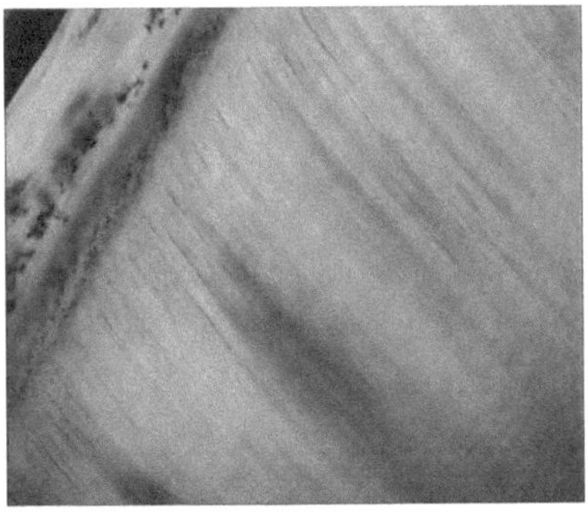

Fig 29: Dental fluorosis with diffuse boundary between cementum and dentin

Figure 30 shows fluorosed teeth with higher grades with increased thickness of Tomes' granular layer.

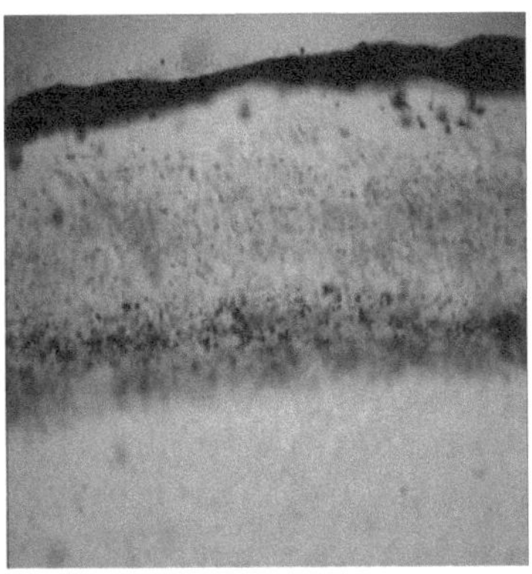

Fig 30: F Teeth – Wider Tom's Granular layer

DF is characterized by opaque, lusterless white patches in the enamel which may become striated, pitted and discolored with a breakdown of mineralized layer shortly after eruption.[62] Opacity results from incomplete crystal growth in enamel in teeth with DF.[63]

As fluorosis becomes more severe, the subsurface enamel throughout the tooth becomes increasingly porous (hypomineralized), with lesions extending into the inner enamel. Reports indicate that in cases of severe fluorotic enamel, significant abrasion occurs on the soft, porous exposed lesions when the well-mineralized surface zone is damaged. This exposure of hypomineralized lesions is a result of substantial changes in the oral environment.(64) Histological examination of teeth from areas of high fluoride concentration showed more alterations in the enamel than that of dentin. This suggests that fluoride affects the processes involved in biomineralization, in general, no matter if the crystal formation and growth occur either in mesenchymal or ectodermally derived mineralized tissues,(63) when higher concentrations of fluoride like 5 ppm can cause mottling and hypoplasia of the enamel and hypomineralized dentin and increased inter-globular spaces Reports indicate that the enamel surface of fluorosed teeth appears highly uneven and rough, displaying cracks and fissures. In the discolored areas, the enamel shows pits of varying sizes, resembling punched lesions on the surface, which expose the underlying porous enamel.(65) Considering the complexity of the biological mineralization process, the exact mechanism leading to DF is not fully understood.(66) A recent study on ground sections of fluorosed teeth reported crescent-shaped hypomineralized areas in enamel and increased inter-globular dentin spaces.(67)

CLINICAL FEATURES

Fluoride is used in community water supplies in the concentration of 0.7-1.2 parts per million (ppm).[68] At this concentration, fluoride is known to reduce dental caries by 50-60% in permanent teeth. It protects against demineralization by inhibiting bacterial enzymes at low levels and promotes remineralization. However, increasing the fluoride concentration to 3 ppm or higher can lead to fluorosis, which may present as either dental or skeletal fluorosis. These adverse effects are typically the result of chronic exposure to high fluoride levels. Dental fluorosis is often the first clinical sign of fluoride toxicity in children. It's important to recognize that the initial changes in enamel, although not easily detectable by an inexperienced observer, signify the first biological indication of excessive fluoride intake during tooth development. Long term intake of fluoride during enamel calcification results in minute white flecks, yellow or brown areas scattered irregularly or streaked over the surface of a tooth, or it may be a condition when the entire tooth surface is of dead paper white colour.[69]

The clinical manifestation of fluoride toxicity may be of two types:

A. Chronic fluoride toxicity: It exerts toxic effects on human beings. It consists of mainly three types of fluorosis, skeletal fluorosis, crippling fluorosis, and dental fluorosis. According to the Merriam-Webster's Collegiate Dictionary (2003), it defines that "Fluorosis is an abnormal condition (as mottling of the teeth) caused by fluorine or its compounds."

B. Acute fluoride toxicity: The acute effects of ingesting large doses of fluoride can occur when a person consumes it as a poison. This may lead to muscle fibre degeneration, deformities in red blood cells, low haemoglobin levels, excessive thirst, headaches, skin rashes, and nervousness. In such cases, a fatal outcome can occur within two to three days [70]

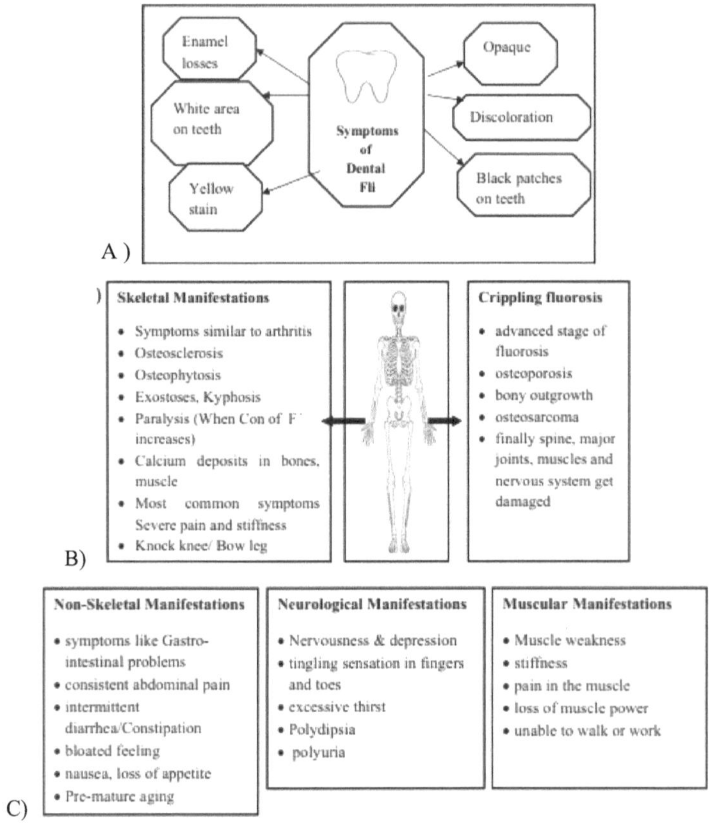

Fig 31: (A) Symptoms of dental fluorosis. (B) Symptoms of skeletal and crippling fluorosis. (C) Symptoms of nonskeletal, neurological, and muscular manifestations.(source: Dwivedi, Shubha & Dwivedi, Naveen. (2021). Environmental aspects of fluoride contamination and treatment of wastewater using hybrid technology.)

Skeletal fluorosis results from the chronic consumption of water with high fluoride levels, as excess fluoride accumulates in skeletal tissues. Symptoms include intermittent joint and bone pain, stiffness in the joints, stomach pain, headaches, and muscular weakness. In addition to fluoridated water, skeletal fluorosis can also arise from the consumption of fluoride-rich foods, inhalation of airborne fluoride, or occupational exposure in various industries and factories. Skeletal fluorosis results in osteosclerosis which causes calcification of bones resulting in impairment of major joints, muscles, spine and nervous system.(69)

FLUOROSIS AT THE TIME OF TOOTH ERUPTION:

Fluoride-induced enamel changes as they appear at the time of eruption range from thin white opaque lines corresponding to the perikymata running across the tooth surface, to an entirely chalky white enamel. [66] In its mildest forms, the porosity is to be found in the outermost enamel only, but the entire tooth surface is involved. With increasing severity, both the depth of enamel involvement and degree of porosity of the enamel increase. Assuming a relatively constant exposure level (most commonly water-borne fluoride), all surfaces of a given tooth will be equally affected [66]

DISTRIBUTION OF FLUOROSIS WITHIN MOUTH:

The changes are symmetrically distributed within the oral cavity, but the severity varies among the different types of teeth. The degree of severity appears in principle to reflect the stage in life at which the various tooth types are formed and mineralized regardless of whether the child is born and reared in a low (0.2) or a higher (1-2 ppm) water fluoride area. The teeth which form and mineralize early in life are those that are least affected, whereas the later in life the teeth mineralize, the more severely they will be affected. According to this concept, exposure to very low fluoride levels will result in only a few teeth exhibiting subsurface porosities to a degree that will be clinically manifested. Dental fluorosis is characterized by increased porosity of the enamel; it is noted that the oral environment may influence the clinical appearance of the enamel once the tooth has erupted into the mouth. However, the degree of post-eruptive modification of the enamel will to some extent also be determined by the degree of hypo-mineralization at the time of eruption. [71]

POST-ERUPTIVE CHANGES IN FLUOROSIS:

In the milder forms of dental fluorosis, mechanical attrition resulting from the use of abrasive tooth paste, will over time cause a "remission" of the fluorotic lesions most likely due to surface enamel removal. The upper incisors are susceptible to such environmental modifications When there is inadequate lip closure, the incisal portion of the central incisors may be exposed to air, leading to prolonged dryness. This can make any porosities more noticeable. As a result, there is a significant tendency for stains to penetrate the exposed enamel, particularly in areas corresponding to the position of the upper lip. Generally, the extent of stain uptake is influenced by the degree of porosity as well as the individual's dietary habits. Therefore, discoloration alone is not a reliable indicator of severity.(64)

In more severe cases of dental fluorosis, the tooth erupts into the oral cavity with a completely chalky white appearance. The degree of porosity (hypomineralization) in these teeth weakens the enamel, causing sections of the superficial enamel to break away. This damage can range from small, scattered pits to larger areas where the outermost enamel is lost. Such loss is particularly common along the incisal edges and cusp tips. In the most severe forms of dental fluorosis, the extent of porosity is so pronounced that a significant amount of the outer enamel may chip off immediately after eruption, exposing the underlying porous enamel, which readily absorbs stains. For an accurate clinical diagnosis of enamel defects, the teeth should be dry, observed with cheek retractors, and examined under good lighting conditions. (71)

CLINICAL FEATURES WITH INCREASING SEVERITY:

A. Mild Fluorosis

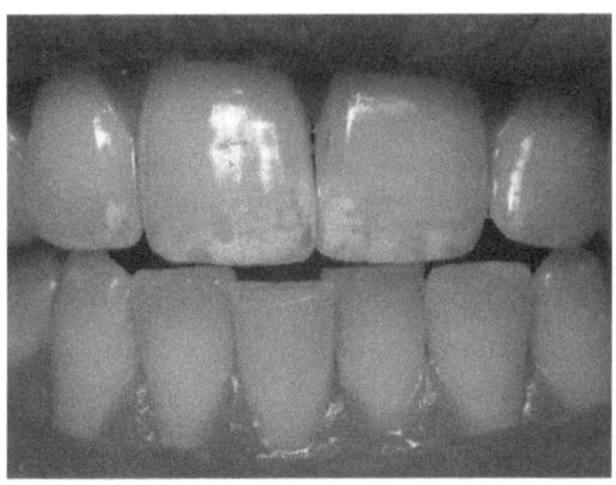

Fig 32: Mild fluorosis

(source: Nakornchai, Siriruk & Hopattaraput, Piyawan & Vichayanrat, Tippanart. (2016). Prevalence, severity and factors associated with dental fluorosis among children aged 8-10 years in Bangkok, Thailand. The Southeast Asian journal of tropical medicine and public health. 47. 1105-1111.)(72)

- The initial indication of dental fluorosis manifests as thin, white striae across the enamel surface. These fine, opaque lines follow the pattern of perikymata and can only be seen after the tooth surface is cleaned. At this early stage, the cusp tips, incisal edges, and marginal areas may also appear completely opaque white, a condition referred to as the "snow cap phenomenon."[73]

- In slightly more affected teeth the white lines become broader and pronounced. Occasional merging of several lines occurs to produce smaller, irregular, cloudy or paper white areas scattered over the surface.

B. Moderate Fluorosis

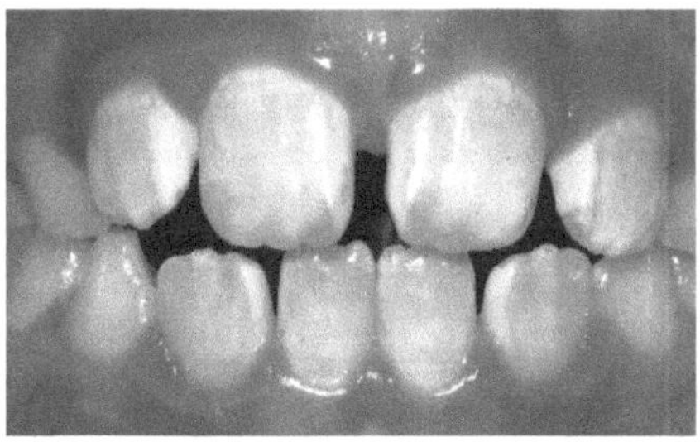

Fig 33: Moderate Fluorosis

(source: Dental fluorosis in Australia [Internet]. Fluoride Free Australia. 2018 [cited 2024 Sep 11])[74]

- With increasing severity, the entire tooth surface exhibits distinct, irregular, opaque or cloudy, white areas. Between these opacities, perikymata lines are often visible.
- In the case of moderate fluorosis, the disturbances result in porosity and over a period of time following eruption, stains are taken up and trapped within the enamel, making these areas more obvious.
- There is a range of dietary chromogenic substances that can be taken up and retained with superficial enamel giving these areas a more distinct appearance. It is not unusual for teeth to erupt with porous, white, opaque areas that may discolour over time.
- Discoloration can occur before eruption; it typically becomes more noticeable after the teeth have erupted.
- Irregular opaque areas may merge, causing the entire tooth surface to appear chalky white. At the time of eruption, this condition can range from a white, opaque tooth that feels relatively hard upon probing to a completely chalky tooth that shows surface damage immediately after eruption.

C. Severe Fluorosis

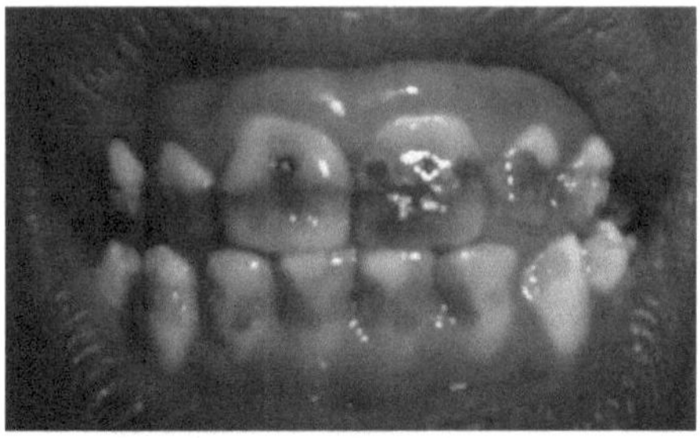

Fig 34: severe fluorosis

(source: Choubisa, Shanti. (2022). Status of chronic fluoride exposure and its adverse health consequences in the tribal people of the scheduled area of Rajasthan, India. 55. 8-30.)[75]

- In more severe form of fluorosis, the impact on the physical properties of enamel is more dramatic. A common sequel to this problem is that at various times following eruption, small areas of enamel are lost spontaneously, giving the appearance of enamel hypoplasia.
- In severe stages, there is a focal loss of outermost enamel. Such enamel defects are usually designated a pits. The pits can vary in diameter and are typically scattered across the surface, although they most commonly appear along the incisal and occlusal halves of the tooth. As the severity increases, these pits can merge to form horizontal bands. In more severely affected teeth, the confluence of the pitted areas leads to larger, corroded sections. [76]
- Ultimately, the most severely fluorotic tooth shows an almost complete loss of surface enamel. This loss can be so significant that only a cervical rim of distinctly opaque enamel remains intact. The rest of the tooth typically displays dark brown discoloration.[77]
- When teeth are highly opaque at the time of eruption, they are very susceptible to attrition and extensive occlusal abrasion is observed in high fluoride areas, even in young individuals.

DIFFERENTIAL DIAGNOSIS OF FLUOROSIS

Fluorosis can be diagnosed through visual examination. Numerous indices have been developed to diagnose, qualify, and quantify the clinical features of dental fluorosis. Differentiating between fluorotic and non-fluorotic disturbances of tooth enamel is essential for developing an appropriate treatment plan. Key risk factors include elevated fluoride levels in drinking water, infant formula mixed with fluoridated water, fluoridated toothpaste, and supplements. Understanding the fluoride content in enamel can aid in diagnosing dental fluorosis. This condition can be distinguished from other enamel defects by examining the color of the enamel, its distribution on the affected teeth, and the extent of unaffected enamel.[(78)]

The diagnosis of dental fluorosis primarily relies on its visual appearance. Confirmation can be achieved by reviewing the patient's medical history, particularly regarding systemic fluoride exposure. In normal enamel, the outer layer has significantly higher fluoride levels compared to the inner layer. The fluoride content in the inner enamel correlates directly with fluoride availability during tooth development, while the outer enamel is influenced by fluoride uptake after eruption.[(73)]

Diagnosing mild dental fluorosis in primary teeth can be challenging due to their thinner enamel and lighter color compared to permanent teeth. Primary teeth generally show less dental fluorosis than their permanent counterparts. This may be attributed to the placenta acting as a barrier to fluoride in fetal circulation, reduced fluoride intake during lactation, or the shorter duration of enamel formation and maturation in deciduous teeth. Additionally, the severity of dental fluorosis tends to increase from anterior to posterior teeth in both types of dentition, with enamel thickness correlating with the severity of the condition.[(79)] It has been observed that the severity of dental fluorosis increases with the age at which enamel formation is completed. For cosmetically important teeth, such as permanent incisors and canines, enamel formation typically concludes by the age of 7. Therefore, concerns about the development of dental fluorosis are primarily focused on the first seven years of life.[(79)]

Differentiation between fluoride and non-fluoride disturbances of dental enamel is a valuable diagnostic step toward an oral epidemiology and public health concern. Several investigators have suggested descriptive indices for classifying other similar non-fluoride enamel opacities. However, endemic prevalence, history of more than optimal fluoride ingestion in drinking water during tooth development, and its bilateral symmetrical pattern are considered as important differentiating features for diagnosing dental fluorosis. (78)

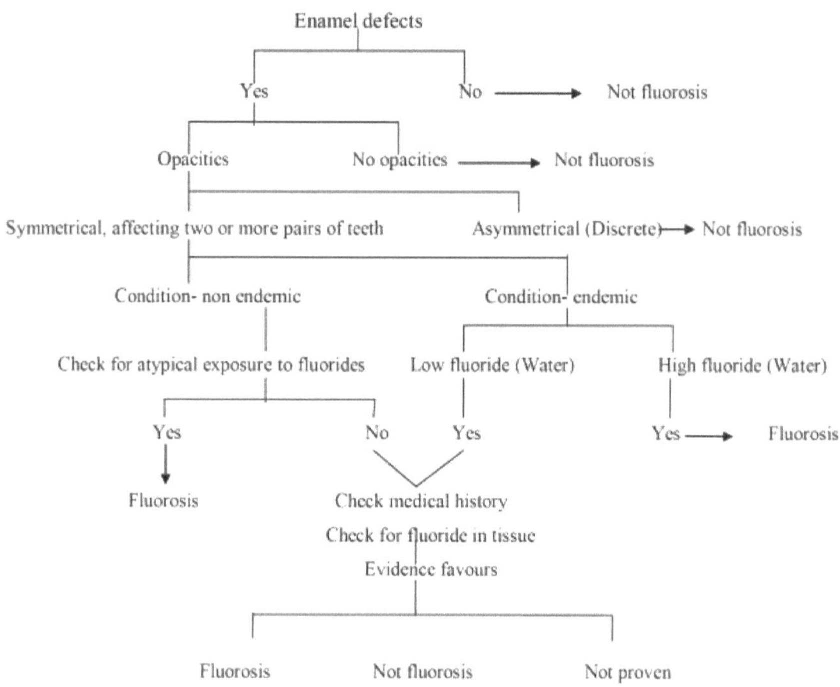

Flow chart showing the sequence recommended for differential diagnosis of dental fluorosis (source: Patidar, Deepika & Sogi, Suma & Patidar, Dinesh & Sharma, Atul & Jain, Mansi & Prasad, Priyanka. (2021). Enlightening Diagnosis and Differential Diagnosis of Dental Fluorosis—A Hidden Entity in a Crowd. Dental Journal of Advance Studies. 9. 10.1055/s-0041-1725218.)

Dental fluorosis can be diagnosed primarily through the appearance of the teeth, particularly the enamel surface. However, other conditions may produce similar changes, making a differential diagnosis essential to exclude these alternatives.[45] Some of the conditions that can be considered in the differential diagnosis of dental fluorosis include:

1. Amelogenesis imperfecta: In this genetic abnormality we can witness structural alterations in the morphology of the tooth hence more or less it might appear similar to that to fluorosis alterations present morphologically.
2. Enamel hypoplasia: This is a condition where there is a deficiency of tooth enamel due to damage or interruption of the enamel-forming cells during tooth development.
3. Hypocalcification: This is a condition where there is a deficiency of calcium in the enamel, leading to a soft and porous enamel that may be more prone to decay.
4. Tetracycline staining: This is a condition where the use of the antibiotic tetracycline during tooth development can lead to a yellow or brown discoloration of the teeth.
5. Trauma: Injury to the teeth can lead to structural changes, including pitting or staining of the enamel surface.

It is quite noteworthy to understand that a proper diagnosis regarding a patient having fluorosis can only be done with the help of taking proper history and noting amount of exposure witnessed along with finding out other potential reasons of having the same. If any person is concerned about any unusual morphological change happening in the tooth then immediate appointment with a dentist should be done and necessary preventive and treatment modalities must be employed.[45]

Features	Dental fluorosis	Amelogenesis imperfecta	Enamel hypoplasia	Dentinogenesis imperfecta	Molar-incisor hypomineralization
Area affected	The entire tooth surfaces often enhanced or near tips of cusps/ incisal edges	Centered in smooth surface of limited extent Hypoplastic—buccal surface Hypomaturation—incisal or occlusal	Localized to the center of the smooth surface	The entire tooth surfaces	Loss of initially formed surface enamel after tooth eruption
Lesion	Show a horizontal striated pattern across the tooth. Bilateral symmetrical Qualitative defect—enamel has normal thickness, but changes in its translucency	Show vertical bands of white, opaque or translucent enamel surface and are round and oval in appearance. Qualitative/ quantitative	Round and oval in appearance. Occurs in the form of pits, grooves Quantitative defect—enamel is of reduced thickness	Affected teeth show distinct translucency and enamel frequently separates from underlying defected dentin	Soft, porous, brittle enamel resembling discolored chalk or old Dutch cheese Qualitative defect—enamel is of normal thickness with a smooth surface
History	High-fluoride level in drinking water in a community with water fluoridation, history of fluoride supplementation	Hereditary/familial pattern	If injury occurs during formative stage of enamel development Incomplete or defective formation of the organic enamel matrix of teeth	Hereditary/familial pattern. Autosomal dominant condition	Systemic alteration during maturation phase of enamel / idiopathic enamel defect with unknown etiology
Demarcation	Diffuse distribution	Clearly differentiated from adjacent normal enamel.	Clearly differentiated from adjacent normal enamel	Clearly differentiated	Sharp demarcation between the affected and sound enamel
Color	Slightly more opaque than normal enamel; "paper white." Incisal edges, tips of cusps may have frosted appearance Does not show stain at the time of tooth eruption	Usually pigmented at the time of eruption; often creamy yellow to dark reddish orange	Brownish discoloration	Bluish to amber brownish	White to yellow or brown in color
Teeth affected	Teeth that calcify slowly (cuspids, bicuspids, second and third molars) Always on homologous teeth Extremely rare on deciduous teeth	Any tooth may be affected Frequent on labial surface of lower incisors Common in deciduous teeth	**Hereditary type**—Both the dentitions are affected **Environmental type**—Either dentition is involved Hutchinson's incisor and mulberry molars are seen (congenital syphilis). Incisors and Premolars (Turner's hypoplasia)	Both the dentitions are involved Deciduous teeth are more affected followed by permanent incisors, first, second and third molars are least affected	Both the dentitions are involved Usually affects permanent molars and incisors
Detection	Often invisible under strong light; easily detected by line of sight tangential to tooth crown	Line of sight perpendicular to tooth surface under strong light	Translucent or opaque	Affected teeth show distinct translucency	Alterations in the translucency of the enamel

(Continued)

Table 2: Difference between dental fluorosis and non-fluoride developmental defects and opacities (source: Patidar, Deepika & Sogi, Suma & Patidar, Dinesh & Sharma, Atul & Jain, Mansi & Prasad, Priyanka. (2021). Enlightening Diagnosis and Differential Diagnosis of Dental Fluorosis—A Hidden Entity in a Crowd. Dental Journal of Advance Studies. 9. 10.1055/s-0041-1725218.)

Features	Dental fluorosis	Tetracycline staining	Pulpal hemorrhage	Internal resorption	Congenital erythropoietic porphyria	Congenital hyperbiliru-binemia and eythroblasto-sis fetalis	Alkaptonuria
Area affected	The entire tooth surfaces or near tips of cusps/ incisal edges	The entire tooth surfaces	The entire tooth surfaces. Anterior teeth are more prone	The entire tooth surfaces	The entire tooth surfaces	The entire tooth surfaces	The entire tooth surfaces
Color	Slightly more opaque than normal enamel; "paper white" to yellowish brown in severe cases	Bright yellow to dark brown	Bluish black	Crown display a pink discoloration (pink tooth of Mummery)	A marked red brown discoloration	Green discoloration	Blue black discoloration
History	High fluoride level in drinking water	Past drug history	History of trauma	Pulpal inflam-mation is usually caused by bacterial invasion	Medical history. An autoso-mal recessive disorder of porphyrin metabolism	Medical history	Medical history. An autosomal recessive metabolic disorder
Mechanism	Successive exposures to high concentration of fluoride during the formative stage of tooth development	Tetracycline and its homologous form complexes with calcium ions on the surface of hydroxyapatite crystals within bone and dental tissues	Hemolysis of the red blood cells releases the hem group to combine with the putrefying pulpal tissue to form black iron sulphide	Vascular resorp-tive process approaches the surface of the crown. Resorbed dentin is replaced by inflamed granula-tion tissue	Increased synthesis and excretion of porphyrins	Deposition of biliverdin (the breakdown product of the bilirubin) and may vary from yellow to green	Defect in the enzyme "homogenti-sate oxidase," homogenti-sate accumu-lates in tissues and blood
Critical time period and the teeth involved	Teeth that calcify slowly (cus-pids, bicuspids, second and third molars). Always on homologous teeth. Extremely rare on decidu-ous teeth	Both the denti-tions are involved. Avoided during pregnancy and in children up to 8 years of age	Both the denti-tions are involved	Both the dentitions	Both the dentitions are involved. In deciduous teeth porphyrin is present in both enamel and dentin while in per-manent teeth only dentin is affected	Mostly decid-uous teeth are affected during the neona-tal period Occasionally, the cusps of the permanent first molar may be affected	Both the dentitions
Detection	Often invisible under strong light; most easily detected by line of sight tan-gential to tooth crown	a bright yellow flu-orescence under UV light	Visible bluish black discoloration.	Visible pink discoloration. On radiograph, a well circumscribed radi-olucent enlarge-ment of the pulp chamber is seen	A red fluores-cence when exposed to a Wood's UV light	Sharp dividing line, sepa-rating green portions from normal colored portions	Bluish black discoloration

Table 3: Difference between dental fluorosis and other tooth discoloration of systemic origin (source: Patidar, Deepika & Sogi, Suma & Patidar, Dinesh & Sharma, Atul & Jain, Mansi & Prasad, Priyanka. (2021). Enlightening Diagnosis and Differential Diagnosis of Dental Fluorosis—A Hidden Entity in a Crowd. Dental Journal of Advance Studies. 9. 10.1055/s-0041-1725218.)

Features	Dental fluorosis	White spot lesion (incipient caries)	Rampant caries
Area affected	The entire tooth surfaces or near tips of cusps/incisal edges	Smooth surfaces near the cervical margin or contact area at proximal surface	Entire tooth surfaces often involved
History	High fluoride level in drinking water or any history of fluoride supplementation	Multifactorial (diet, oral hygiene, etc.) Posteruptive etiology	Multifactorial (diet, oral hygiene) Improper feeding practice
Mechanism	Successive exposures to high concentration of fluoride during the formative stage of tooth development	Change in tooth enamel due to loss of the structure in the oral environment/ demineralization of tooth enamel	Demineralization of tooth enamel and progression of lesion to dentin and even pulp
Lesion	Show a horizontal striated pattern across the tooth. Bilaterally symmetrical	The subsurface porosity caused by demineralization gives a milky white appearance	Single tooth or even bilateral teeth involvement
Demarcation	Diffuse distribution over the surface of varying intensity	Visible on drying the tooth surface	Visible cavitated brown/black lesions.
Teeth involved	Teeth that calcify slowly (cuspids, bicuspids, second and third molars). The mandibular incisors are least affected. Always on homologous teeth. Extremely rare on deciduous teeth	Any tooth may be affected depending on the local attack of acid Both the dentitions are involved	Proximal surface of mandibular anterior teeth which are immune to decay are also involved Both the dentitions are involved
Detection	Often invisible under strong light; detected by line of sight tangential to tooth crown	Seen under fiberoptic light at an angle to the tooth surface	Visible cavitated brown /black lesions
Color	Slightly more opaque than normal enamel; "paper white," incisal edges, tips of cusps may have frosted appearance No staining at the time of tooth eruption	Usually pigmented at the time of eruption; often creamy yellow to dark reddish orange	Dark brown to blackish in appearance

Table 4 : Difference between dental fluorosis and dental caries

(source: Patidar, Deepika & Sogi, Suma & Patidar, Dinesh & Sharma, Atul & Jain, Mansi & Prasad, Priyanka. (2021). Enlightening Diagnosis and Differential Diagnosis of Dental Fluorosis—A Hidden Entity in a Crowd. Dental Journal of Advance Studies. 9. 10.1055/s-0041-1725218.)

A comprehensive clinical history, along with the distribution of the condition on the affected tooth or within the dentition, the pattern of lesions, color, and the method of detection, are key diagnostic criteria for distinguishing dental fluorosis from non-fluoride related tooth discolorations.

DIAGNOSIS

Fluorosis is important to measure because it is a condition that reflects the level of fluoride exposure during enamel formation and this condition should be monitored regularly *(O'Mullane et al., 2016).* When fluorosis is found to be prevalent in a community, it is essential to implement measures to reduce fluoride intake among children with developing teeth. However, fluctuations in the prevalence of fluorosis can also result from the varying methods used to measure the condition. For instance, a study focusing on the public health significance of fluorosis will have different criteria compared to one examining the detailed biological effects of fluoride. Accurate diagnosis of fluorosis is essential, especially for distinguishing it from other enamel defects caused by various factors such as malnutrition, celiac disease, rickets, and premature birth *(Browne et al., 2005).* These differing criteria have led to the development of multiple indices and assessment methods for enamel fluorosis. Despite the abundance of these indices, several studies have evaluated the agreement among examiners using them, but newer measurement techniques have received comparatively less attention.(80)

MEASUREMENT INDICES

Several indices were developed to measure dental fluorosis in the 20th century. These include fluorosis specific indices such as Dean's Index (DI); the Thylstrup and Fejerskov (TF) Index; the Total Tooth Surface Index (TSIF); and the Fluorosis Risk Index (FRI). Non-specific descriptive indices such as the Developmental Defects of Enamel (DDE) index have also been used to record fluorosis.

Direct clinical examination and imaging techniques are the most common methods used to measure fluorosis.(80)

A. Direct Clinical examination

Clinical examination is commonly utilized because it is quick, simple, cost-effective, and allows for the assessment of all tooth surfaces, along with tactile evaluation. However, this method has its drawbacks, including variations in examination techniques, lighting conditions, potential examiner bias, and issues with examiner reliability. Furthermore, direct clinical assessments heavily rely on the cooperation of the subjects, particularly when multiple indices are used simultaneously.[80]

Measurement of Dental Fluorosis:

a) A visual analogue scale(VAS) by *Vieira et al* 2005.

b) Quantitative Light Fluorescence Assessment of Dental Fluorosis by *Pretty et al* 2006.

c) Quantitative Light Fluorescence and Polarised white light assessment of dental fluorosis—*Pretty et al* 2012.

1. VISUAL ANALOGUE SCALE (VAS)

This scale was developed by *Vieira et al.* in 2005 to address the limitations of previous indices that did not utilize a continuous scale. Recognizing that photographs are a valid method for measuring fluorosis, a Visual Analog Scale (VAS) was created based on aesthetic perceptions of these images, employing a 100-millimeter (mm) continuous scale. The scale is marked at each end, with the left labeled "best you can imagine" and the right labeled "worst you can imagine," representing the spectrum of enamel surface quality. Five photographs showcasing varying severities of dental fluorosis served as indicators for this scale. The main advantages of the VAS for dental fluorosis over the ordinal scales for dental fluorosis (such as TFI,DI,TSIF) are the continuity of the scale, its simplicity and its precision. It uses visual indicators to measure dental fluorosis. These indicators guide examiners through the scale and help them use it precisely. The benefits of using a VAS over other indices are the continuity of the scale and its simplicity of use.The primary criticism of the VAS is its lack of specific criteria for scale points, making it susceptible to examiner bias. While the scale includes photographs representing various severities of dental fluorosis as indicators, the assessment remains highly subjective. This subjectivity can complicate examiner training and calibration efforts.[80]

2. QUANTITATIVE LIGHT FLUORESCENCE (QLF)

This was described by *Pretty et al* in 2006. This scale was developed to address certain limitations associated with traditional photography, particularly the challenge of assessing dental fluorosis in relation to other enamel defects. The phenomenon of personal thresholding particularly at low levels of fluorosis severity with differences in the application of diagnostic criteria and the variability in inter and intra-examiner agreement are also issues of concern with traditional photography. Training of examiners will also be costly and complex. Therefore, the need for assessment of dental fluorosis by an automated grading system. The principle of QLF is to compare changes in fluorescence between sound enamel and 'unsound enamel' (loss of fluorescence intensity in areas of enamel hypomineralization). Images were assessed by computer software. However, specular reflection is a cofounder. however, the main limitation of QLF is the inability to differentiate mineral loss as a result of fluorosis or other forms of enamel defects. Other features such as caries, restorative material or extrinsic staining also interfere with the QLF analysis.(80)

3. POLARIZED WHITE LIGHT IMAGES

In 2012, *Pretty et al.* proposed another technique namely a dual imaging system, which is a combined method between fluorescent imaging and polarized white light. Polarization provides better images which eliminate the specular reflection for assessment using an automated grading system. Additional advantages of using this dual camera system are the ability to facilitate the use of an automated system and minimize the need for photographic training. the technique being easy to operate and well accepted by the subjects. This system is relatively new and is ambitious in fluorosis assessment. Its cost-effectiveness is also unknown.(80)

B. IMAGING TECHNIQUES

To address the limitations of clinical examination, imaging techniques have been developed to create a permanent record of the enamel surface for assessing fluorosis. The use of clinical photographs for measuring dental fluorosis gained prominence in the 21st century, as previous indices were subjective and susceptible to bias. Clinical photographs can be captured during examinations and graded remotely. This method not only allows for archiving and tracking longitudinal changes but also facilitates scoring by multiple examiners, enables remote assessment, and enhances the creation of training sets for examiner calibration.

The main advantages of using images are

1. it allows blinding of the examiner(s), which minimize examiner bias, and archiving of the images allows repeated measurement by multi examiners at a location remote from the clinical examination sight.
2. Permanent record provided by photographs can also be kept for longitudinal assessment, future measurement using different indices and training of examiners.

The disadvantages of imaging methods are

1. They are technique sensitive, and variation can be introduced by the technique used to take the image, the camera equipment and the quality of the image produced.
2. There is an issue with specular reflection caused by the ring flash used to provide adequate lighting. This can result in over reporting prevalence of dental fluorosis. This is mainly due to the appearance of reflections from the flash that might mimic the appearance of white spot lesions.
3. It is only suitable for anterior teeth, photographic access to posterior teeth being poor.

While several researchers have suggested multi-view techniques to address these issues *(Wong et al., 2005),* some surfaces or parts of surfaces may still be overlooked, even with multiple perspectives *(Golkari et al., 2011).* This oversight can lead to an underreporting of fluorosis prevalence compared to a whole-mouth examination. Additionally, utilizing photographs increases the overall cost of the study compared to relying solely on clinical examination. Imaging techniques in assessing fluorosis can be divided into conventional and digital photography. In the early adoption of imaging techniques for assessing fluorosis, conventional photography was commonly utilized. Although photographic methods have advanced from conventional film transparencies to digital images, some researchers still prefer conventional photography to facilitate data comparison with earlier studies that employed standardized. [80]

Recently, many researchers have reported using digital photography for fluorosis assessment. The advantages of digital photography include the ability for examiners to evaluate the quality of images immediately after capture, allowing for retakes if the image is unsatisfactory. It also enables zooming and adjustments to achieve the best image quality, as opposed to being restricted by a fixed barrel lens *(Golkari et al., 2011).* Furthermore, digital photography can better accommodate patient confidentiality and can be stored in digital systems. Images are produced instantaneously without the need for developing negatives or printing. However, the downsides include the higher cost of equipment and the need for a skilled photographer experienced in using digital cameras.[(80)]

INDICES

Quantifying dental fluorosis is a crucial step in epidemiological studies and dental public health, serving as a key tool for determining the incidence, prevalence, and severity of the condition. This assessment helps to establish the fluorosis status or health status of individuals in relation to other population groups, providing insights into the relative status of the population. Measuring dental fluorosis is essential for surveillance, research, and treatment planning. An effective index for measuring any condition should be sensitive, easy to understand, and reliable. In the 20th century, the various indices used for measurement of dental fluorosis are:[9]

1.Dean's Index- 1934
2.Community Fluorosis Index-1946
3.Thylstrup-Fejerskov Index-1978
4.Tooth surface Index of Fluorosis -1984
5.Fluorosis Risk Index-1990
6. The developmental defects of enamel index-1982
7.Indian Council of Medical Research (ICMR) Index -2013

1. DEAN'S INDEX [81]

Dean provided a standard classification system for clinical conditions as described by *McKay* on 2000 subjects in endemic areas of six states in USA. It was first described in 1934 and was later modified in 1942. The index was developed to gain an understanding of the relationship between fluoride concentrations in drinking waters and mottled enamel. It emphasizes the aesthetic aspect of dental fluorosis. It has become the most widely accepted classification system for dental fluorosis affecting two or more teeth. In cases where two teeth are not equally affected, the less affected tooth is scored. Dean's Index remains popular due to its simplicity and its capacity to facilitate comparisons with numerous earlier studies. In their assessment of examiner reliability for this index, *Kumar et al.* demonstrated good to excellent agreement beyond chance, with the level of agreement on the presence or absence of fluorosis using Dean's definition ranging from 92% to 97%.

Shortcoming of Dean's Index –

- Single score is given to a tooth rather than, a separate score to each tooth surface. Hence differences in the severity of fluorosis in different tooth surfaces cannot be ascertained.
- Questionable diagnostic category (score 0.5) in Dean's Index is difficult to define and interpret precisely.
- The distinctions between some of the diagnostic categories in Dean's system are unclear, imprecise or lack sensitivity. (81)

Although Dean's index has been in use for over 50 years, it is not without shortcomings. Dean's classification —questionable has caused a lot of confusion, though, Dean intended the questionable category to be used in cases where the examiner was unsure as to whether opacities should be defined as normal/ very mild. It is also considered that DI is not able to give sufficient information on the distribution of dental fluorosis within the dentition especially with its lowest score- the questionable score. DI scores are ordinal and thus creating problems in data analysis and it is argued that DI scores are not sensitive enough. The index cannot discriminate between severe forms of dental fluorosis. Consequent to these limitations, other scoring systems have been developed. (81)

Classification And weight	Original criteria (Dean, 1934)	Modified criteria (Dean, 1942)
Normal 0	The enamel presents the usual translucent semi-vitriformtype of structure. The surface is smooth and glossy and usually of a pale creamy white color.	The enamel presents the usual translucent semi-vitriform type of structure. The surface is smooth, glossy and usually of a pale creamy white color.
Questionable 0.5	Slight aberrations in the translucency of normal enamel, ranging from a few white flecks to occasional white spots, 1 to 2 mm in diameter	The enamel discloses slight aberrations from the translucency of normal enamel, ranging from a few white flecks to occasional white spots. This classification is utilized in those instances where a definite diagnosis of the mildest form of fluorosis is not warranted and a classification of "normal" not justified.
Very Mild 1.0	Small, opaque, paper-white areas are scattered irregularly or streaked over the tooth surface. It is principally observed on the labial and buccal surfaces, and involves less than 25% of the tooth surfaces of the particular teeth affected. Small pitted white areas are frequently found on the summits of the cusps. No brown stain is present in the mottled enamel of this classification.	Small, opaque, paper-white areas scattered irregularly over the tooth but not involving as much as approximately 25% of the tooth surface. Frequently included in this classification are teeth showing no more than about 1-2 mm of white opacity at the tips of the summits of the cusps of the bicuspids or second molars.
Mild 2.0	The white, opaque areas on the surfaces of the teeth involve at least half of the tooth surface. The surfaces of molars, bicuspids, and cuspids subject to attrition show thin white layers worn off and the bluish shades of underlying normal enamel. Faint brown stains are sometimes apparent, generally on the upper incisors.	The white opaque areas in the enamel of the teeth are more extensive but do not involve as much as 50% of the tooth.
Moderate 3.0	No change is observed in the form of the tooth, but generally all of the tooth surfaces are involved. Surfaces subject to attrition are definitely marked. Minute pitting is often present, generally on the labial and buccal surfaces. Brown stain is frequently a disfiguring complication. It must be remembered that the incidence of brown stain varies greatly indifferent endemic areas, and many cases of white opaque mottled enamel, without brown stain, are classified as "moderate" and listed in this category.	All enamel surfaces of the teeth are affected, and surfaces subject to attrition show marked wear. Brown stain is frequently a disfiguring feature.
Moderately Severe	Macroscopically, a greater depth of enamel appears to be involved. A smoky white appearance is often noted. Pitting is more frequent and generally observed on all the tooth surfaces. Brown stain, if present, is generally deeper in hue and involves more of the affected tooth surfaces.	
Severe 4.0	The hypoplasia is so marked that the form of the teeth is at times affected, the condition often being manifest in older children as a mild pathologic incisal occlusal abrasion. The pits are deeper and often confluent. Stains are widespread and range from a chocolate brown to almost black in some cases	It Includes teeth formerly classified as "moderately severe" and "severe". All enamel surfaces are affected, and hypoplasia is so marked that the general form of the tooth maybe affected. The major diagnostic sign of this classification is the discrete or confluent pitting. Brown stains are widespread and teeth often present a corroded like appearance.

Table 5: clinical criteria and scoring for deans Index

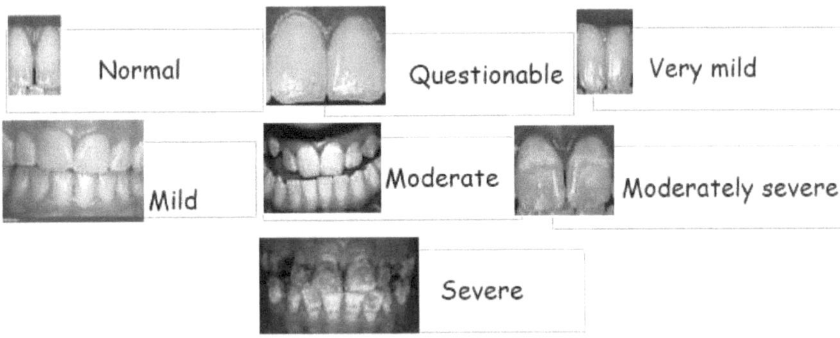

Fig 35 : Criteria for Dean's Classification System for Dental Fluorosis (1934)(source: an assessment of dental fluorosis in school children of vallioor union in tirunelveli district Saifullah Mohamed Ramlath Sabura* 1 Somasundaram Muthalagi2 and Magil Inbaraj Delighta Mano Joyce. World Journal of Pharmaceutical Research Volume 8, Issue 10, 1471-1479.)

2. COMMUNITY FLUOROSIS INDEX[81]

Trendly H Dean in 1946 devised a method of calculating the prevalence and severity of fluorosis in a group or community which he termed as 'Community fluorosis Index' (CFI). This gave an indication of the public health significance of the fluorosis

CFI= n×w /N

Where n= number of individual in each category

w= the weighting for each category

N= total population

Public health significance of CFI index

Range of Scores for Community Fluorosis Index	Public Health Significance
0.0 - 0.4	Negative
0.4 - 0.6	Border line
0.6 - 1.0	Slight
1.0 - 2.0	Medium
2.0 - 3.0	Marked
3.0 - 4.0	Very marked

Table 6 : Public Health Significance of Community Fluorosis Index Scores, as Defined by Dean (1946) (source: Horowitz HS. Indexes for measuring dental fluorosis. J Public Health Dent. 1986 Fall;46(4):179-83. doi: 10.1111/j.1752-7325.1986.tb03139.x. PMID: 3465956.

3. THYLSTRUP AND FEJERSKOV INDEX (TFI)

The *Thylstrup and Fejerskov* developed an index in order to refine, modify and extend the original concepts established by Dean. The primary aim was to develop a more sensitive classification system for recording enamel changes associated, with increasing level of fluoride in water. The basis of TFI is the classification scale, closely to the histological changes that occur and fluoride content found in the enamel. A 10-point ordinal scale is used to classify enamel changes associated with increasing fluoride exposure. As originally proposed, facial and occlusal surfaces were scored with different criteria. From 1988, onwards the scoring of facial surface was recommended for TFI. The sensitivity of TFI comes from its 9 stages reflecting the histopathology and fluoride content in the enamel. It is sensitive, easy to understand, reliable and at the most outstanding for evaluating the severity of fluorosis. TFI had an excellent reproducibility despite its extended scale, was suitable to categorize mild forms of dental fluorosis withease, due to drying of teeth before scoring and had clear description and discrimination of the categories in the lower end of the index [66]

Critics of TFI

The TFI seems more appropriate than Dean's Index for use in clinical trials or analytical epidemiologic studies, primarily because teeth are dried and fluorosis can be identified in its milder forms. This feature of the TFI is a particular advantage when potential fluoride effects are small, or when the exposure may be wide spread.(82) On comparing the Dean and TF indexes, latter was more detailed and sensitive, because it was based on biological aspects.(83)

Score	Score original criteria (Thylstrup and Fejerskov, 1978)	Modified criteria (Fejerskov *et al.* 1988)
0	Normal translucency of enamel remains after Prolonged air-drying.	The normal translucency of the glossy, creamy-white enamel remains after wiping and drying of the surface.
1	Narrow white lines located corresponding to the perikymata.	Thin white opaque lines are seen running across the tooth surface. The lines correspond to the position of the perikymata. In some cases, a slight "Snowcapping" of cusps/incisal edges may also be seen.
2	Smooth surfaces More pronounced lines of opacity which follow the perikymata. Occasionally confluence of adjacent lines. Occlusal surfaces Scattered areas of opacity < 2 mm in diameter and pronounced opacity of cuspal ridges.	The opaque white lines are more pronounced and frequently merge to form small cloudy areas scattered over the whole surface. "Snowcapping" of incisal edges and cusp tips is common.
3	Smooth surfaces Merging and irregular cloudy areas of opacity. Accentuated drawing of perikymata often visible between opacities. Occlusal surfaces Confluent areas of marked opacity worn areas appear almost normal but usually circumscribed by a rim of opaque enamel	Merging of the white lines occurs, and Cloudy areas of opacity occur spread over many parts of the surface. In between the cloudy areas, white lines can also be seen
4	Smooth surfaces The entire surface exhibits marked opacity or appears chalky white. Parts of surface exposed to attrition appear less affected. Occlusal s urfaces Entire surface exhibits marked opacity. Attrition is often pronounced shortly after eruption.	The entire surface exhibits a marked opacity or appears chalky white. Parts of the surface exposed to attrition or wear may appear to be less affected.
5	Smooth and occlusal surfaces Entire surface displays marked opacity with focal loss of outermost enamel (pits) < 2 mm in diameter	The entire surface is opaque, and there are round pits (focal loss of the outermost enamel) that are less than 2 mm in diameter.
6	Smooth surfaces Pits are regularly arranged in horizontal bands < 2 mm in vertical extension. Occlusal surfaces Confluent areas < 3 mm in diameter exhibit loss of enamel. Marked attrition	The small pits may frequently be seen merging in the opaque enamel to form bands that are less than 2 mm in vertical height. In this class are also included surfaces where the cuspal rim of facial enamel has been chipped off, and the vertical dimension of the resulting damage is less than 2 mm
7	Smooth surfaces Loss of outermost enamel in irregular areas involving < 1/2 of entire surface. Occlusal surfaces Changes in the morphology caused by merging pits and marked attrition.	There is a loss of the outermost enamel in irregular areas, and less than half the surface is so involved. The remaining intact enamel is opaque.
8	Smooth and occlusal surfaces: Loss of outermost enamel involving >1/2 of surface.	The loss of the outermost enamel involves more than half the enamel. The remaining intact enamel is opaque.
9	Smooth and occlusal surfaces Loss of main part of enamel with change in anatomical appearance of surface.Cervical rim of almost unaffected enamel is often noted.	The loss of the major part of the outer enamel results in a change of the anatomical shape of the surface/tooth. A cervical rim of opaque enamel is often noted.

Table 7: clinical criteria and scoring for TF Index

Source: Thylstrup A, Fejerskov O. Clinical appearance of dental fluorosis in permanent teeth in relation to histologic changes. Community Dent Oral Epidemiol. 1978 Nov;6(6):315–28.

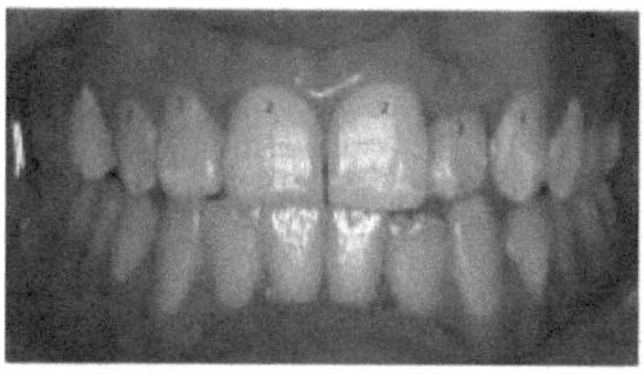

Figure 1A. Dental Fluorosis classification (score 2).

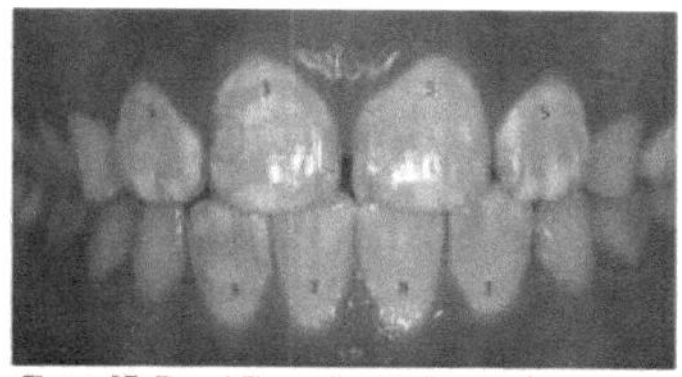

Figure 1B. Dental Fluorosis classification (score 3 and 5). Enamel loss in the tooth 12, 11, 21 and 22.

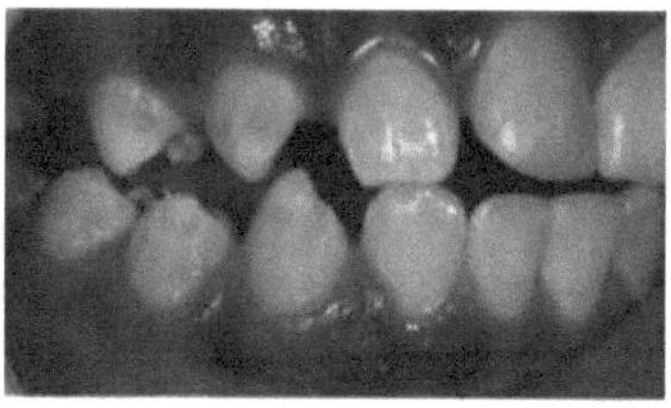

Figure 2A. Dental Fluorosis classification (score 4 and 5). Enamel loss in the teeth 16, 44 and 45.

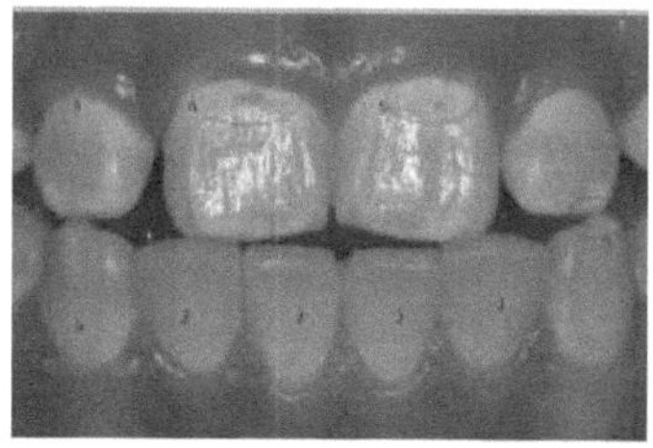

Figure 2B. Dental Fluorosis classification (score 2, 3, 5 and 6). Enamel loss in the teeth 11, 21 and 33.

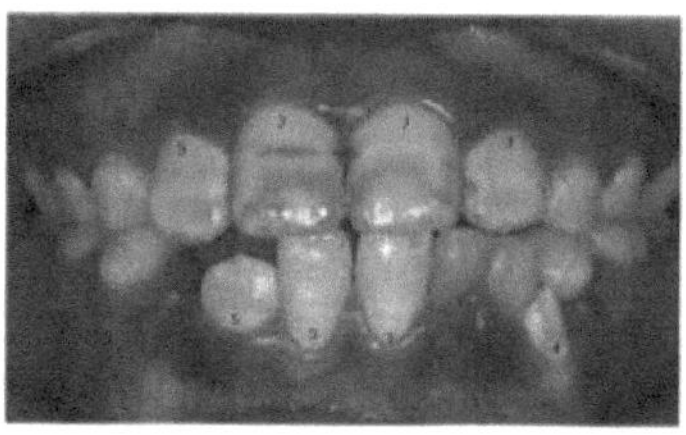

Figure 3A. Dental Fluorosis classification (score 4, score 5 and score 7). Enamel loss in the teeth 12, 11, 21, 22, 31, 41, 42.

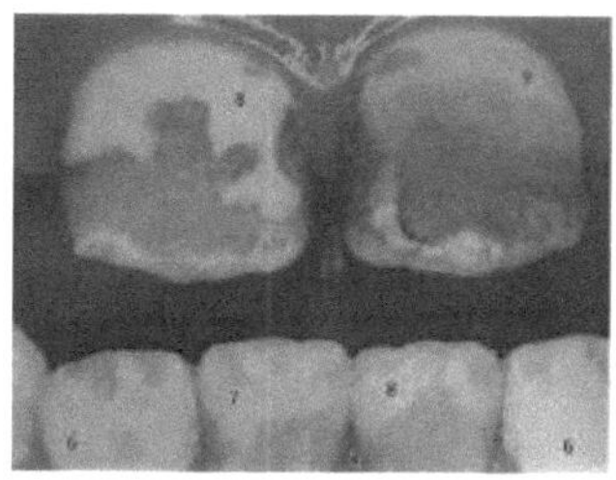

Figure 3B. Dental Fluorosis classification (score 8 in the tooth 11 and the score 9 in the tooth 21).

Source: Thylstrup A, Fejerskov O. Clinical appearance of dental fluorosis in permanent teeth in relation to histologic changes. Community Dent Oral Epidemiol. 1978 Nov;6(6):315–28.(66)

4. TOOTH SURFACE INDEX OF FLUOROSIS (TSIF)

Proposed by *Horowitz et al.* in 1984, this index was designed to address some of the shortcomings of Dean's Index. It allows for a separate assessment of cosmetic fluorosis, which includes discoloration, staining, or pitting on surfaces visible to others. According to the authors, each unrestored tooth surface receives a separate score. Anterior teeth are assigned two scores (for the labial and lingual aspects), while posterior teeth receive three scores (for the buccal, lingual, and occlusal aspects). The TSIF distinguishes between different levels of pitting and differentiates between staining alone and staining accompanied by pitting. Developed and utilized by researchers at the National Institute of Dental Research in the USA, this index is more sensitive than Dean's Index for detecting mild forms of fluorosis

The tooth surface index of fluorosis has identified seven types.[84]

Score	Criteria
0	Enamel shows no evidence of fluorosis.
1	Enamel shows definite evidence of fluorosis, namely, areas with parchment-white color that total less than one-third of the visible enamel surface. This category includes fluorosis confined only to incisal edges of anterior teeth and cusp tips of posterior teeth ("snow capping").
2	Parchment-white fluorosis totals at least one third of the visible surface, but less than two thirds.
3	Parchment-white Fluorosis totals at least two thirds of the visible surface.
4	Enamel shows staining in conjunction with any of the preceding levels of fluorosis. Staining is defined as an area of definite discoloration that may range from light to very dark brown.
5	Discrete pitting of the enamel exists, unaccompanied by evidence of staining of intact enamel. A pit is defined as a definite physical defect in the enamel surface with a rough floor that is surrounded by a wall of intact enamel. The pitted area is usually stained or differs in color from the surrounding enamel.
6	Both discrete pitting and staining of the intact enamel exit.
7	Confluent pitting of the enamel surface exists. Large areas of enamel may be missing, and the anatomy of the tooth may be altered. Dark-brown stain is usually present.

Table 8: Descriptive criteria and scoring system for Tooth Surface Index

(source :Horowitz HS, Driscoll WS, Meyers RJ, Heifetz SB, Kingman A. A new method for assessing the prevalence of dental fluorosis--the Tooth Surface Index of Fluorosis. J Am Dent Assoc. 1984 Jul;109(1):37-41. doi: 10.14219/jada.archive.1984.0268. PMID: 6611361).(84)

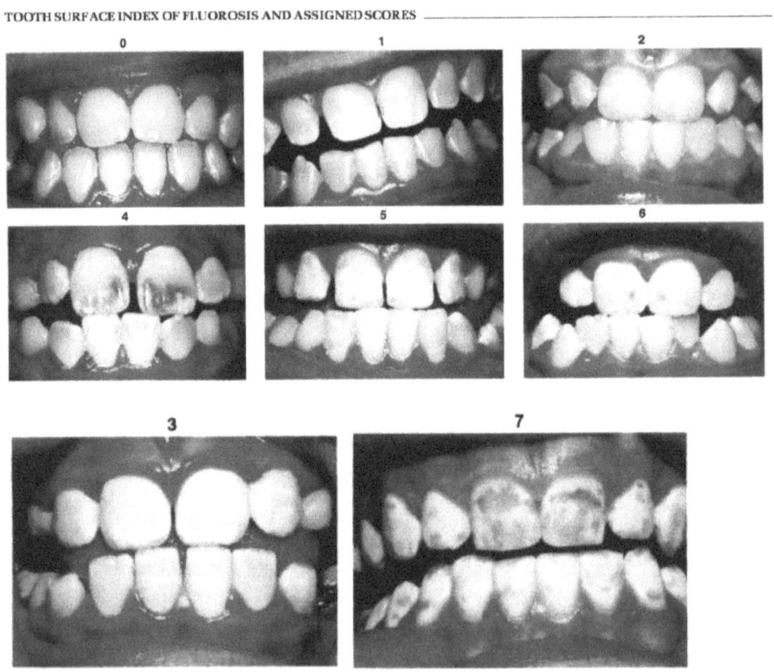

Fig 37 (source: Horowitz HS, Driscoll WS, Meyers RJ, Heifetz SB, Kingman A. A new method for assessing the prevalence of dental fluorosis--the Tooth Surface Index of Fluorosis. J Am Dent Assoc. 1984 Jul;109(1):37-41. doi: 10.14219/jada.archive.1984.0268. PMID: 6611361).(84)

Critics of TSIF

Examiner reliability may be of more concern than with Dean's Index or the modified TFI because of the larger number of assessments to be made. Lingual surfaces are more difficult to visualize than buccal surfaces, which also adds to the concern about examiner reliability.[84]

In comparing the 3 main indices (DI, TFI, TSIF), Pereira and Moreira concluded that if the same measuring methods are used, the three fluorosis indices had similar prevalence, however they suggested appropriate indications for each as follows:

1). Dean 's index: for comparative studies between prevalence and those found in the decades of the 30's and 40's.

2). T-F Index: for clinical studies or analytical epidemiological studies.

3). TSIF: for studies in which an esthetic basis is desired for defining case and also it may be used where risk factors are identified or when the teeth may not be cleaned or dried.(9)

5. FLUOROSIS RISK INDEX [85]

This was proposed by *Pendrys* in 1990 and can been used in Analytical Epidemiological studies. It was designed to permit a more accurate identification of risk factors of enamel fluorosis and developed to allow for the identification of the time during tooth maturation at which exposure was most likely to have been experienced.

This index divides the enamel surfaces of teeth in the secondary dentition into 2 groups of surface zones:

i.) Classification 1-Enamel surface zones that begin formation during the first year of life

ii.) Classification 11- Enamel surface zones that begin formation between the third to sixth year of life

The areas assigned to classification 1 are the incisal edges of the mandibular central and lateral incisor and maxillary central incisors, and the occlusal tables of mandibular and maxillary first molars. These surfaces are at risk of fluorosis if fluoride exposure occurs during the specified time. For classification 11, the areas include the cervical 3rd of the incisors, middle 3rd of the canines and the occlusal table, incisal 3rd and middle 3rd of the bicuspids and 2nd molars in both maxillary and mandibular arches.

Fluorosis Risk Index Enamel Surface Zone Assignments

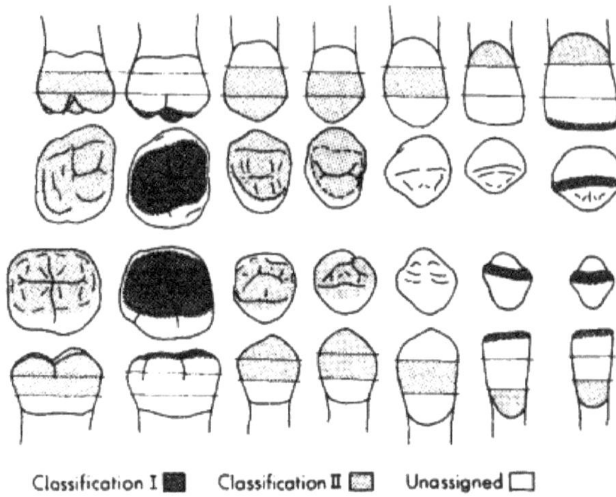

Fig 38: Fluorosis Risk index enamel surface zone assignments

(source: Pendrys DG. The fluorosis risk index: a method for investigating risk factors. J Public Health Dent. 1990;50(5):291–8.)

Criteria for scoring fluorosis

Negative finding

Score = 0

A surface zone will receive a score of O when there is absolutely no indication of fluorosis being present. There must be a complete absence of any white spots or striations, and tooth surface coloration must appear normal.

Questionable finding

Score = 1

Any Surface zone that is questionable as to whether there is fluorosis present (i.e., white spots, striations, or fluorotic defects cover 50 percent or less of the surface zone) should be scored as 1.

Score = 7

Any surface zone that has an opacity that appears to be non-fluoride opacity is scored as 7

Positive findings

Score = 2

A smooth surface zone will be diagnosed as being positive for enamel Fluorosis if greater than 50 percent of the zone displays, parchment while striations typical of enamel fluorosis. Incisal edges and occlusal tablets will be scored as positive for enamel fluorosis if greater than 50 percent of that surface is marked by the Snow capping typical of enamel Fluorosis.

Score = 3

A surface zone will be diagnosed as positive for severe fluorosis if greater than 50 percent of the zone displays pitting, staining, and deformity, indicative of several Fluorosis.

Surface zone excluded

Score = 9

A surface zone is categorized as excluded (i.e. not adequately visible for a diagnosis to be made) when any of the following conditions exist;

Incomplete eruption

Rule 1: If a tooth is in proximal contact but the occlusal surface is not parallel with existing occlusion, the occlusal two thirds of the tooth is scored, but the Cervical one third is recorded as excluded

Rule 2: If a tooth is erupted, but not yet in contact, the Incisal/occlusal edge is scored, but all other surfaces are recorded as excluded.

Orthodontic appliances and bands

Rule 1: If there is an orthodontic band present on a tooth only the occlusal table or Incisal edge should be scored

Rule 2: If greater than 50 % of the surface zone are banded, the subject should be excluded from the examination.

Surface crowned or restored

Rule: Surface zones that are replaced by either a crown or restoration covering greater than 50% of the surface zone should be recorded as excluded.

Gross plaque and debris Rule: Any subjects with gross deposits of plaque or debris on greater than 50% of the surface zones should be excluded from examination.

Critics of Fluorosis risk index

The index is complex, both from a biological perspective and in its application. Acceptable levels of examiner reliability may be difficult to establish due to this complexity.[85]

6. DEVELOPMENTAL DEFECTS OF ENAMEL

This was proposed in 1982 by Commission on Oral Health, Research and Epidemiology arising from a lack of a well-defined and internationally accepted classification of enamel defects. The index was designed to promote use of standard terminology, simplicity and to provide an effective system for recording enamel defects in large studies. The first version was, however complicated and difficult to analyze thus, *Clarkson and O'Mullane* [86] suggested a modified and simplified version of the index that has now been widely adopted

DDE is now the most currently and widely used index in the United Kingdom to study enamel defects. DDE index is descriptive but not specific for fluorosis thus when the objective of the study is to find the prevalence/ severity of fluorosis, DDE index might not be suitable. However, *Sabieha* and *Rockfound* a good correlation between the index and TF index and concluded that either will yield broadly comparable results where it may be expected that fluoride induced opacities will form a significant proportion of all enamel defects found.[9]

Defect	*Code*
Normal	0
Demarcated opacity	1
Diffuse opacity	2
Hypoplasia	3
Other Defects	4
Combinations	
Demarcated and diffuse	5
Demarcated and hypoplasia	6
Diffuse and hypoplasia	7
All three defects	8

Table 9: Classification of Defects According to the Modified DDE Index

(Source: Ruiz, Luciana & Maya, Rafael & D'Alpino, Paulo & Atta, Maria & Svizero, Nádia da. (2013). Prevalence of Enamel Defects in Permanent Teeth of Patients with Complete Cleft Lip and Palate. The Cleft palate-craniofacial journal: official publication of the American Cleft Palate-Craniofacial Association. 50. 394-399. 10.1597/11-200.) (87)

In this classification system, the defects are categorized as hypoplasia, demarcated opacity, and diffuse opacity, which considers the following.

Hypoplasia

Hypoplasia is a defect involving the surface of the enamel and is associated with a reduced thickness of enamel. It can occur in the form of pits, grooves, or large areas of missing enamel (Suckling, 1989).

Pits: single and multiple, shallow or deep, scattered or aligned, or horizontally arranged on the surface of the tooth.

Grooves: single and multiple, narrow or wide (maximum 2 mm)

Partial or complete absence of enamel over a considerable area of dentine; the affected enamel may be translucent or opaque

Demarcated Opacity

This is characterized by an alteration in the translucency of the enamel, variable in degree. The defective enamel is of normal thickness with a smooth surface. It has a clear boundary with the adjacent normal enamel and can be white, cream, yellow, or brown. The lesions vary in extent, position on the tooth surface, and distribution in the mouth (Suckling, 1989).

Diffuse Opacity.

This defect involves an alteration in the translucency of the enamel, variable in degree. The defective enamel is of normal thickness and at eruption has a smooth surface and is white. It can have a linear, patchy, or continuous distribution, but there is no clear boundary with the adjacent normal enamel. Part or all the tooth surface can be affected (Suckling, 1989).

Other Defects.

Those not found in categories of demarcated opacity, diffuse opacity, or hypoplasia include staining caused by tetracycline.

Combination of Defects.

There can be a presence of opacity and hypoplasia on the same tooth surface.[87]

Basic Type of DDE	Subtype of DDE
Demarcated opacities (DEO)	demarcated opacities (white/cream)
	Demarcated opacities (yellow/brown)
Diffuse opacities (DIO)	Diffuse opacities lines/patchy
	Diffuse opacities confluent
	Confluent/patchy stain gloss of enamel
Hypoplasia (EH)	Hypoplasia pits
	Hypoplasia missing enamel
Discolouration	

Table 10: The DDE modified Index

(source: Guerra, Fabrizio & Mazur, Marta & Corridore, Denise & Capocci, Mauro & Ottolenghi, Livia. (2014). Developmental Defects of Enamel : an increasing reality in the everyday practice. Senses and Sciences. 1. 87-95. 10.14616/sands-2014-3-8795.)

7. INDIAN COUNCIL OF MEDICAL RESEARCH (ICMR) INDEX

To address fluorosis, the Indian Council of Medical Research (ICMR) established a task force with four subgroups, one of which focused on dental fluorosis. This subgroup recommended the development of grading and identification criteria for dental fluorosis that health professionals could use with basic training. Consequently, the ICMR Index for Dental Fluorosis was introduced in 2013. The index characterizes dental fluorosis on an ordinal scale of 0-3. In addition, the guidelines for the diagnosis of teeth were also given by ICMR.(89)

Guidelines for screening using ICMR index for fluorosis.(90)

(i) All 28 permanent teeth to be examined.

(ii) Third molar, if present to be excluded because it erupts at different periods or may not erupt at all.

(iii) Tooth should be examined in natural light with a mirror and probe.

(iv) All surfaces of teeth should be examined giving importance to labial surfaces of anterior teeth and buccal surfaces of posterior teeth.

(v) During examination, a probe should be passed on the affected tooth to find out whether it is a smooth surface or has any pit or destruction because of fluorosis.

(vi) Teeth should not be dried with air prior to examination, but only wiped by cotton or gauze.

(vii) Each tooth should be examined and graded individually based on surface texture and color.

(viii) An individual must be graded based on minimum two teeth having highest severity grade.

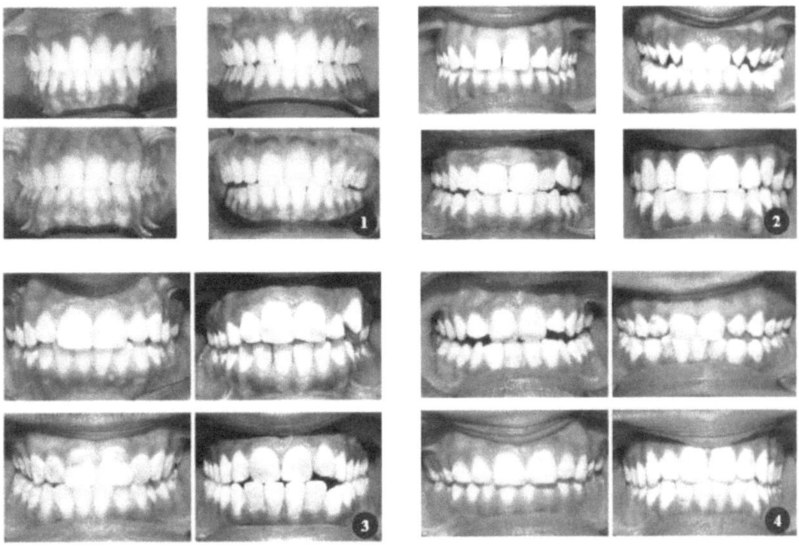

Fig. 1. Grade 0 - Normal appearance of enamel in children with normal teeth. **Fig. 2.** Grade 1- Mild fluorosis cases among the children examined. **Fig. 3.** Grade 2 - Moderate fluorosis cases among the children examined. **Fig. 4.** Grade 3 - Severe fluorosis cases among the children examined.

Fig 39: ICMR Index for dental fluorosis (2013) (source: Goyal A, Verma M, Toteja G, Gauba K, Mohanty V, Mohanty U, et al. Validation of ICMR index for identification of dental fluorosis in epidemiological studies. Indian J Med Res. 2016;144(1):52.)

ICMR index for dental fluorosis

- Grade 0 (Normal): Enamel surface appears smooth, glossy, translucent, creamy white/pale in colour
- Grade 1 (Mild): Enamel surface showing extensive chalky white opaque areas in two or more teeth
- Grade 2 (Moderate): Enamel surface showing brownish yellow or brown colour horizontal lines frequently disfiguring bands or patches on two or more teeth
- Grade 3 (Severe): Enamel surfaces showing brown colour with pitted, discrete or confluent, eroded or destroyed structure on two or more teeth

Index/ Authors	Advantages	Disadvantages
Dean's Index (DI) (Dean, 1934)	Simple to use; accepted at global level; long track record of use supported by literature; allow historical comparison with old studies; recognized by World Health Organization for use in oral health surveys basic method; teeth are examined wet - more relevance to concerns in a public health context (Elwood *et al.* 1994).	Only measure the two most severely affect teeth, does not allow measurement of fluorosis on different tooth surfaces; no information about location of affected teeth; the diagnostic category for 'questionable' in the classification is unclear and lacks precision; the index lacks sufficient precision to distinguish different degrees of fluorosis; teeth are examined wet-may overlook minor opacities (Horowitz, 1986; Clarkson 1989; Rozier, 1994).
Thylstrup- Fejerskov (TF) Index (Thylstrup and Fejerskov, 1978)	Record histological changes that occur in dental fluorosis based on an ordinal scale which allows sufficient precision to distinguish different degrees of fluorosis; TF index has been validated clinically and histologically; TF index is as commonly used as Dean's Index and is particularly favoured in European studies; teeth are examined dry - improve diagnostic sensitivity (Pretty *et al.*, 2006).	Difficult to standardize tooth dryness; the effect of drying may reveal a short period of changes which have less aesthetic or public health importance; the criteria for score 1 and 2 describe only very minor changes. (Clarkson, 1989).
Developmental Defect of Enamel (DDE) Index (FDI, 1992)	Detail measurement that includes a broad range of defects with information on the distribution and location; teeth are examined wet - more relevance to concerns in a public health context. (Elwood *et al.* 1994).	Teeth are examined wet-may overlook minor opacities; time-consuming to conduct due to large information collected.
Tooth Surface Index of Fluorosis (TSIF) (Horowitz *et al.*, 1984)	A score is given to all surfaces instead of individual teeth; the index improves diagnostic sensitivity for fluorosis in severe categories; the index permits a distinction between discrete pitting and more advance confluent pitting and staining alone and staining with pitting; the index is useful especially in populations where severe fluorosis is prevalent; teeth are examined wet - more relevance to concerns in a public health context.	Scoring all surfaces may increase surface-to-surface variation between examiners; scoring lingual and hard to see surfaces may reduce examiner consistency; possibility of losing data on occlusal surfaces because of restorations; teeth are examined wet-may overlook minor opacities (Rozier, 1994).
Fluorosis Risk Index (FRI) (Pendrys, 1990)	The scoring system of different zones of a tooth surface; allow identification of risk factors of fluorosis; useful for analytical epidemiology studies because it allows identification of age-specific exposure to fluoride sources and development of enamel fluorosis (Rozier, 1994).	The index is complex for its biological perspective and application; suitable to estimate of relative risk of fluorosis rather than fluorosis prevalence; the many surface zones to be scored may lead to the possibility of misclassification and increase surface variation both within and between examiners (Rozier, 1994).

Table 11: The different types of indices along with their advantages and disadvantages

(Source: Mohd nor NA. Methods and indices in measuring fluorosis: A review. Arch Orofac Sci. 2017.

MANAGEMENT OF FLUROSIS

Prevention is the best approach to the management of dental fluorosis, but when severely fluorosed teeth are aesthetically objectionable, restorative management may be indicated. In milder cases with dis-coloration, tooth-whitening procedures or micro-abrasion may be beneficial.

1. PREVENTIVE MEASURES

De-fluoridation Dental fluorosis is best prevented by avoiding excessive fluoride intake during the late secretory and maturation phases of enamel, a period that extends to 3-4 years of age for permanent anterior teeth. Thus, drinking water in areas with endemic dental fluorosis should be de-fluoridated to contain appropriate fluoride levels". Depending on the climatic conditions, fluoride concentration of 0.7-1.2ppm is generally considered appropriate, and the World Health Organization has set the upper limit at 1.5ppm.(91)

Under hot climatic conditions in such countries as Senegal, Sudan and Saudi Arabia, however, exposure to fluoride levels that would be regarded as 'sub-optimal' has resulted in severe dental fluorosis in some children. in determining the appropriate fluoride level, a balance has to be struck between the anti-caries effect of fluoride and the cosmetic disadvantage of dental fluorosis.

2. CONTROLLED USE OF FLUORIDE IN PREVENTIVE DENTISTRY

Consideration should be given to fluoride ingestion from drinking water and other sources before prescribing fluoride supplements so as not to overburden the tissue fluids with excessive fluoride during the period of tooth formation. Daily fluoride ingestion of 0.05-0.07mg/kg body weight during enamel formation is generally regarded as optimal." or as an upper limit". (92)

SUPERVISION OF THE USE OF FLUORIDE TOOTHPASTE IN CHILDREN

The widespread use of fluoride toothpaste is sometimes regarded as one of the major risk factors for the increase in the prevalence of dental fluorosis in areas with fluoride-deficient public water supplies. This is partly because children swallow a significant part of the toothpaste they use to minimize the amount of toothpaste swallowed, tooth brushing by children aged below 5 years should be supervised: the amount of toothpaste used each time should be related to their age and/ body weight and they should be encouraged to spit out the toothpaste after brushing.[93]

3. MANAGEMENT OF FLUOROSIS BY THERAPEUTIC MEASURES

Discoloration of teeth is the primary reason patients seek treatment for fluorosed teeth. This discoloration may result from white opacities due to enamel hypomineralization. The absorption of extrinsic stains into the porous subsurface enamel can lead to discoloration, which may appear yellowish, light brown, dark brown, or black. [Figures 40 and 41].

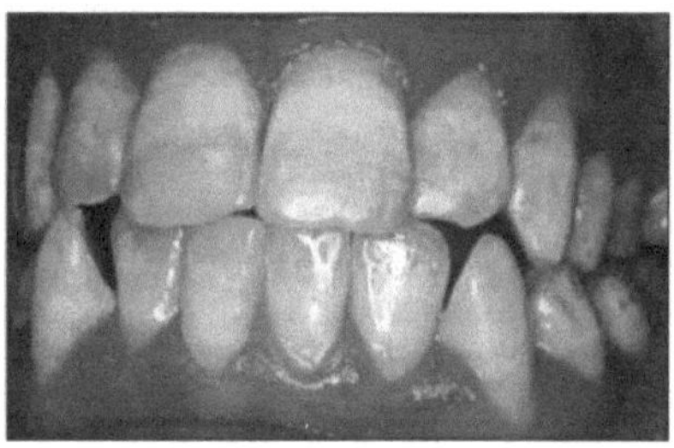

Fig 40: Opaque white anterior teeth with staining (TFI = 4)(Source: Akpata ES. Therapeutic management of dental fluorosis: A critical review of literature. Saudi J Oral Sci. 2014 Jun;1(1):3.)

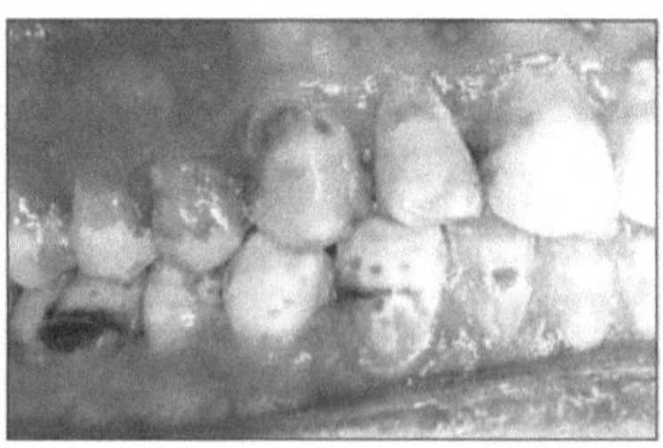

Fig 41: Fluorosed teeth with yellow stains and loss of surface enamel (TFI = 5-8)(Source: Akpata ES. Therapeutic management of dental fluorosis: A critical review of literature. Saudi J Oral Sci. 2014 Jun;1(1):3.)

To restore the natural white creamy appearance of the enamel, the tooth may be bleached, or the subsurface porosities and entrapped extrinsic stains can be removed through microabrasion or macroabrasion. If the subsurface porosities are too deep to be effectively treated with microabrasion without causing hypersensitivity or compromising the aesthetic appearance, the enamel surface may be covered with porcelain or resin composite veneers. In cases where more than 50% of the surface enamel has been lost due to fluorosis, the remaining enamel may not provide adequate support for adhesive bonding, necessitating a crown for the fluorosed tooth. It has been observed that more severe enamel fluorosis correlates with deeper subsurface porosities.[66] Thus, *Akpata* suggested that mild fluorosis with T-F score of 1-2 should be managed by bleaching, as the subsurface porosities may be sufficiently superficial for the entrapped extrinsic stains to be removed by the bleaching agent.[10] To facilitate the penetration of the bleaching agent into the subsurface porosities of the enamel, the hypermineralized surface enamel may be etched with phosphoric acid. [66]

Akpata suggested in 2001 that for T-F scores of 3-4, microabrasion should be considered, as the subsurface porosities might be so deep that the entrapped extrinsic stains are not easily accessible to bleaching alone. Microabrasion can effectively remove both the subsurface porosities and the trapped extrinsic stains. Since the loss of surface enamel in a fluorosed tooth is often a result of post-eruptive occlusal trauma, a tooth with a TFI of 4 may potentially progress to a T-F score of 5 if it experiences significant occlusal trauma.[66] Therefore, in order to be as conservative as possible in the management of dental fluorosis, it has been suggested that micro abrasion should first be tried on teeth with TFI = 4, and if ineffective, the tooth should then be treated by laminate veneer.[10] For teeth with TFI = 5-7 veneering is suggested, but if more than 50% of enamel surface has been lost, as in teeth with TFI = 8-9, the fluorosed tooth should be crowned. The management options suggested for discolored fluorosed teeth are, therefore, bleaching, microabrasion (or macroabrasion), veneering and crowning. [66]

1. BLEACHING

According to McCloskey, the first attempt to eliminate fluorosis stains was carried out by Dr. Walker Kane, Colorado Springs, in 1916. He rubbed the teeth with muriatic acid (HC1). He first applied the flame of an alcohol torch then he finally settled for the acid alone. In 1942, Younger stated that the use of an acid caused enamel decalcification and tended to make the treated teeth more susceptible to caries. He advised the use of a bleaching solution of 5 ml of 30% H202 and 1 ml of anesthetic ether. The reaction is accelerated by applying a heated instrument on the tooth surface. [15]

McInnes added chloridric acid to Younger's solution and presented his famous formula: a fresh solution of 5 ml of hydrochloric acid (36%), 5 ml of hydrogen peroxide (30%), and 1 ml of anesthetic ether. It is applied directly to the tooth; the patient's gums, mucosa, and face obviously being protected. Neutralization is accomplished by a mixture of sodium bicarbonate and distilled water or with a 5.25% sodium hypochlorite solution. To help remove the stains, Bailey and Christen and Colon modified Mclnnes's method by using a fine cuttle disk after applying the bleaching solution. Finally, McCloskey suggested the use of a 18% solution of hydro- chloric acid made by diluting 36% HC1 with equal parts of distilled water which, when applied directly to the tooth, would eliminate stains.[15]

Discolored, mildly fluorosed teeth have been treated by in-office or at-home bleaching or a combination of both. Hydrogen peroxide (35%) and carbamide peroxide (10%) are the commonly used bleaching agents. High concentrations (e.g. 35% hydrogen peroxide) of the bleaching gel are used for in-office bleaching. Before applying the gel directly to the teeth, they are isolated and cleaned. The action of the gel can be enhanced using a halogen or light-emitting diode (LED) curing light. Multiple in-office bleaching sessions may be needed to achieve the desired results. To help the bleaching agent penetrate the subsurface porosities of the fluorosed tooth, the hypermineralized surface layer may be conditioned with 37% phosphoric acid. After in-office bleaching, at-home bleaching can be continued until the desired shade is reached.[94]

Additionally, the application of calcium sucrose phosphate gel has been suggested to enhance the appearance of fluorosed teeth affected by white opacities. The process involves cleaning the tooth and etching it with 37% phosphoric acid for 2 minutes, followed by the application of 2% sodium fluoride for 4 minutes.

Finally, a 40% calcium sucrose phosphate gel is applied.

Enamel blemishes caused by dental fluorosis may also be addressed using Wright's protocol.(95) The fluorosed tooth is first cleaned with prophylaxis paste. The enamel surface is then etched with 35% phosphoric acid to enhance the penetration of sodium hypochlorite, which serves as the bleaching agent. The bleaching process may be repeated until the desired shade is achieved. After bleaching, the enamel pores are sealed with a low viscosity resin composite to prevent further stain absorption into the subsurface porosities. The fluorosed teeth selected for this bleaching technique were classified within grades 1-4 of the TSIF.

The method proposed by *Belkir* et al. in 1991 is quite similar to Wright's protocol. In this technique, enamel is etched with 12% hydrochloric acid to eliminate post-eruptive calcified surface enamel and expose microcavities that contain stains. This is followed by the application of pure sodium hypochlorite to effectively remove the stains. Finally, the chemically opened microcavities are filled with resin composite. The effectiveness of the night guard vital bleaching technique (NGVBT) for removing dental fluorosis stains was studied in 2003. [41]

Different concentrations of carbamide peroxide and hydrogen peroxide were used:

- 20% carbamide peroxide (Opalescence/Ultradent, USA),
- 10% carbamide peroxide (NuProgold/Dentsply, USA)
- 7.5% hydrogen peroxide (Day White/Discus Dental, USA)[41]

The teeth of the subjects in the double blind clinical trial, had TSIF of 1-3, while patients with TSIF of 4-5 were excluded. The three bleaching products were effective in bleaching the discolored teeth, the 20% carbamide peroxide being most effective after 1 week of bleaching.

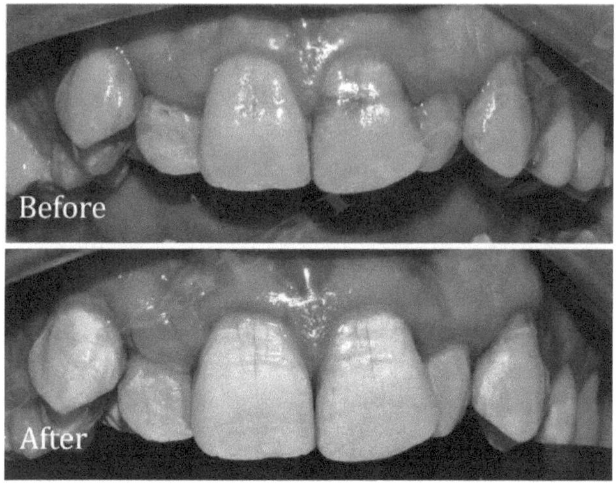

Fig 42: Bleaching of Fluorosed Teeth (Source: Katarmal DB. Dental Bleaching for Fluorosis of Teeth [Internet]. [cited 2024 Sep 6].

2) MICROABRASION

Microabrasion is the controlled removal of superficial stain from enamel. The technique is used for removing stains due to mild-to-moderate fluorosis. Micro-abrasion first evolved from a technique previously carried out by Walker Kane in 1916 but first described by *Mc'Closkey* and modified by *Croll and Cavanaugh.* Microabrasion is frequently used in conjunction with bleaching to effectively eliminate fluorosis stains. It is considered the treatment of choice for mild fluorosis (TFI = 1-3), though it can also be attempted in cases of moderate fluorosis (TFI = 4). The discolored tooth is first etched with phosphoric acid, after which a thick mixture of pumice and 18% hydrochloric acid is applied to abrade the tooth surface. This process removes both the enamel porosities and the entrapped extrinsic stains.(14)

To mitigate tooth hypersensitivity following microabrasion, amorphous calcium phosphate (ACP) is applied. Additionally, a complex of casein phosphopeptide (CPP) and ACP has shown potential in reducing the opaque white discoloration associated with enamel fluorosis by promoting remineralization. A combination of microabrasion and at-home bleaching is recommended, along with chair-side restoration of the superficial enamel microstructure. In this approach, microabrasion targets the removal of the hypermineralized, white-colored superficial enamel layer, while at-home bleaching focuses on eliminating the extrinsic stains trapped within the subsurface porosities. One case made use of Opalustre (Ultradent) for microabrasion, then sodium fluoride to minimize hypersensitivity, followed by at-home bleaching with 10% carbamide peroxide for 2 weeks. Finally, the enamel surface was reshaped with fine-grit diamond to recreate natural enamel appearance.[14]

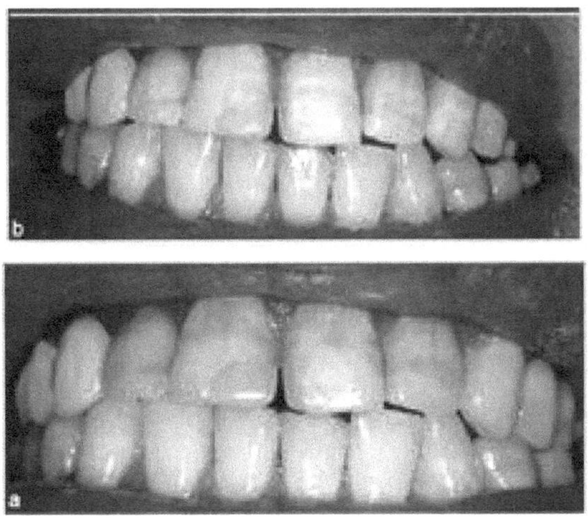

Fig 43 : Microabrasion of maxillary anterior teeth with mild fluorosis (TFI = 3): (a) - Preoperative, (b) - Postoperative.)(Source: Akpata ES. Therapeutic management of dental fluorosis: A critical review of literature. Saudi J Oral Sci. 2014 Jun;1(1):3.)

The abrasion of enamel prisms, combined with the erosion caused by acid in the abrasion slurry, leads to a compacted surface devoid of enamel prisms, which alters its optical properties. This phenomenon is sometimes referred to as the "abrasion effect" or "enamel glaze." Additionally, surface irregularities resulting from extensive exposure of deep-seated porosities may be noticeable after treating severe fluorosis. Therefore, it can be concluded that microabrasion is only recommended for mild fluorosis treatment. Faster techniques for removing fluorosis stains, often called macroabrasion, have been proposed. These methods include using fine-grit diamond points at high speed or sandpaper discs at low speed. While effective for addressing deep-seated fluorosis stains, these methods may also lead to excessive removal of tooth tissue.[14]

3) LAMINATE VENEERS AND FULL CROWNS

Laminate veneers are used to manage severe dental fluorosis, especially where there has been surface enamel loss. It has been suggested that teeth with TFI = 5-7 should be restored with laminate veneers. Likewise, cases with TFI = 4 in which microabrasion or macroabrasion have not been successful. The veneer may be made of porcelain or resin composite.(10)

Since adhesive bonding to enamel yields more predictable results than bonding to dentin, laminate veneers are not recommended when over 30% of the labial enamel has been lost. Significant enamel loss makes it challenging to avoid placing the veneer preparation margins in dentin, which can increase the risk of postoperative sensitivity. Consequently, it is advised that teeth with a TFI of 8-9 be crowned, as these fluorosed teeth have lost more than 50% of their enamel. Porcelain laminate veneers are known for their excellent track record, providing outstanding appearance and predictability while being biocompatible. In contrast, resin composite laminate veneers have several drawbacks, including marginal staining, material loss, and gingival irritation.(10)

TOOTH PREPARATION

Preparation of severely fluorosed teeth for laminate veneers follows the usual general principles. Nevertheless, certain special considerations need to be borne in mind. Display of incisal enamel would be unaesthetic. Therefore, the window type of labial enamel preparation, should be avoided. Rather, the incisal bevel preparation is preferable.

After removing 0.3-0.5 mm of labial enamel during preparation of a severely fluorosed tooth for a laminate veneer, there may be residual enamel discoloration. The enamel stain should be removed by in-office bleaching, using 25-38% hydrogen peroxide or 35-40% carbamide peroxide. (10) Teeth that mineralize later in life are more severely impacted by fluorosis, resulting in darker blemishes, particularly on premolars. When preparing only the anterior teeth for veneers, if the premolars appear very dark, it is advisable to bleach the posterior teeth before selecting the shade for the veneers. Alternatively, the shade can be made progressively lighter from the posterior to the anterior teeth. (14)

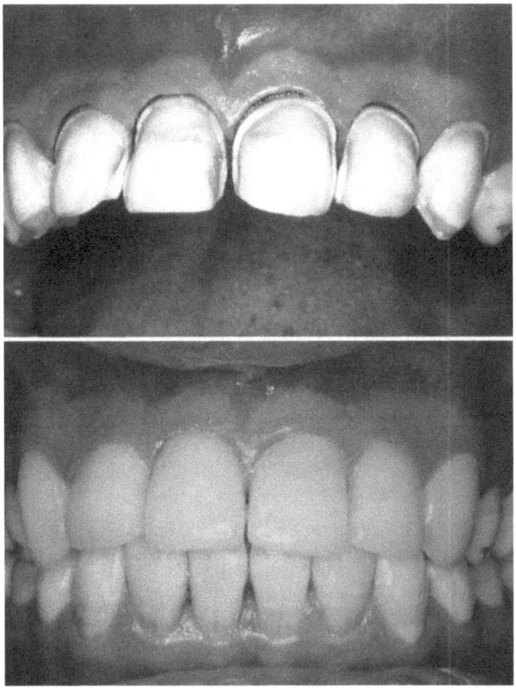

Fig 44: (a) Fluorosed teeth prepared for laminate veneers and (b) after cementation of the veneers (Source: Akpata ES. Therapeutic management of dental fluorosis: A critical review of literature. Saudi J Oral Sci. 2014 Jun;1(1):3.)

EFFECT OF FLUOROSIS ON ETCHING OF HUMAN ENAMEL

Fluorosed enamel is characterized by an outer hypermineralized layer that is resistant to acid, alongside areas of subsurface hypomineralization that contain more porous enamel. These pores are filled with water and enamel secretory proteins, which remain due to the impact of excessive fluoride levels on ameloblasts. (97)The depth of etch of non-fluorosed teeth is affected not only by the type and concentration of the acid etchant, but also by the etching time and the chemical composition of the enamel. Because the fluorapatite in the hypermineralized surface layer of fluorosed teeth is more resistant to acid dissolution than the hydroxyapatite in non-fluorosed teeth, it has often been suggested the etching time of fluorosed enamel be doubled.(98)

The depth of etch of fluorosed enamel with TFI 1–3 is not significantly different from that in non-fluorosed teeth and generally increases with etching time. When enamel with TFI 4 is etched for 15 s, the depth of etch is extremely shallow, but at an etching time of 30 s, the depth of etch is not significantly different from that obtained for teeth with TFI 1–3. In contrast, the depth of etch obtained for enamel with TFI 5 and 6 correlates poorly with the etching time. Fluorosed teeth produce typical etching patterns, unrelated to the severity of fluorosis.

When teeth with TFI 5–6 are etched for 30–45 s, the subsurface insoluble organic network becomes evident, but disappears and typical etching patterns re-appear when the etching time is increased to 60–90 s. Therefore, in clinical practice, etching of mildly fluorosed teeth with white lines or discrete opaque areas (TFI 1–3) should be same as for non-fluorosed teeth (TFI-0). However, the etching time of moderately fluorosed teeth with completely opaque enamel (TFI-4) should, at least, be doubled. For severely fluorosed teeth with pitted or focal loss of surface enamel (TFI-5–6), the hypermineralized surface layer together with the organic network should be ground away before etching the subsurface enamel in the same manner as mildly fluorosed teeth; alternatively, the etching time should be prolonged (at least 90 s) to remove both the hypermineralized surface layer. (99)

There are three options available when etching teeth with TFI 5–6 for adhesive restorations. The first option is to grind away the hypermineralized surface layer together with the organic network to expose the subsurface layer for etching. The second option is to etch for a short duration (30–45 s) to expose the organic network and remove the material with an organic solvent, thus producing an enamel surface possibly resembling type II etching pattern. The third option is to etch for a long duration (at least 90 s) to remove both the hypermineralized surface layer and organic network as well as etch the subsurface enamel, all in one step. The choice between these three options would depend on the one that produces the highest bond strength with adhesive restorations. (99)

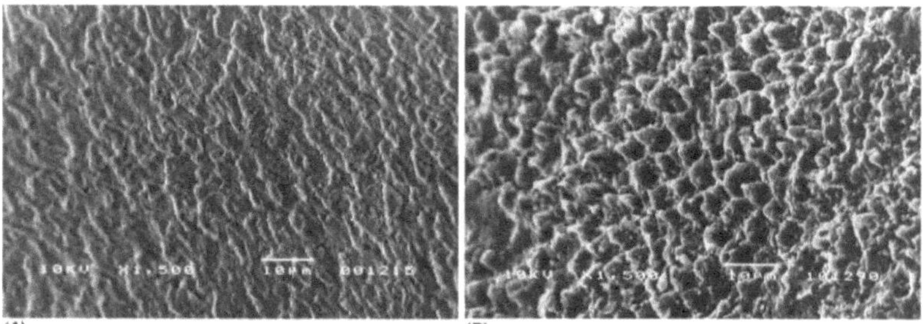

(A) (B)

Fig 45: SEM photomicrograph showing: (a) slight surface roughening of enamel specimen at TFI_2 etched for 15 s (original magnification _1500); (b) accentuated type II etching pattern of enamel specimens at TFI_2 etched for 90 s (original marginal magnification _1500).(source: Al-Sugair MH, Akpata ES. Effect of fluorosis on etching of human enamel. J Oral Rehabil. 1999 Jun;26(6):521–8.)

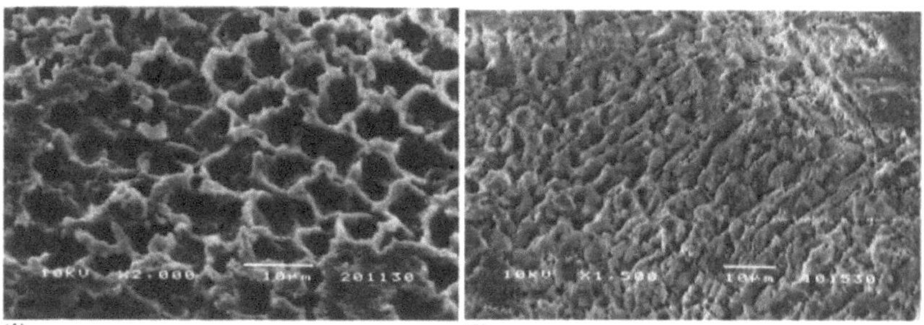

(A) (B)

Fig 46: SEM photomicrograph showing: (a) type I etching pattern on enamel specimen at TFI_1 etched for 30 s (original magnification _2000); (b) rather indistinct etching pattern of enamel specimen at TFI_5 etched for 30 s (original magnification _1500). (source: Al-Sugair MH, Akpata ES. Effect of fluorosis on etching of human enamel. J Oral Rehabil. 1999 Jun;26(6):521–8.)

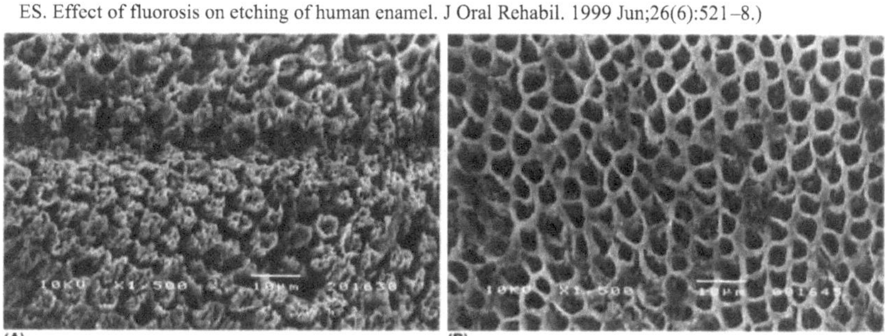

(A) (B)

Fig 47: SEM photomicrograph showing: (a) types I and II etching patterns with generalized surface pitting on enamel specimens with TFI_6 etched for 30 s (original magnification _1500); (b) insoluble organic network or mesh seen on enamel specimen with TFI_6 etched for 45 s (original magnification _1500). (source: Al-Sugair MH, Akpata ES. Effect of fluorosis on etching of human enamel. J Oral Rehabil. 1999 Jun;26(6):521–8.)

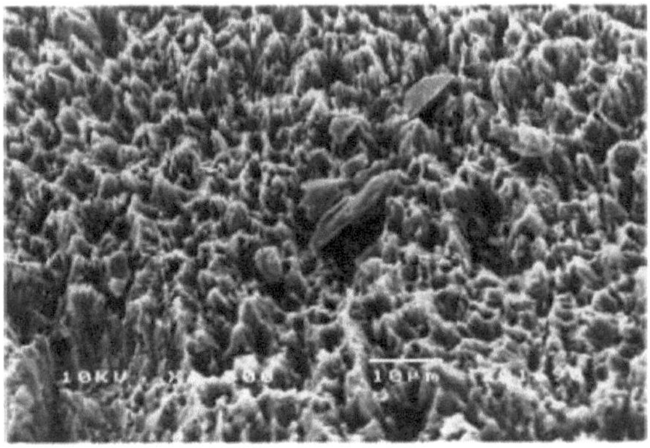

Fig 48: SEM photomicrograph showing re-appearance of normal etching patterns on enamel specimens with TFI_6 etched for 90 s (original magnification _1500). (source: Al-Sugair MH, Akpata ES. Effect of fluorosis on etching of human enamel. J Oral Rehabil. 1999 Jun;26(6):521–8.)

BONDING PROTOCOLS TO FLUOROSED TEETH

ENAMEL

Resin cements are utilized for bonding laminate veneers and crowns in the aesthetic treatment of severe fluorosis. Studies have shown that when the hypermineralized surface enamel is left intact, the bond strength is negatively impacted by fluorosis. (100) On the other hand, bond strength was unaffected by severity of fluorosis when surface enamel was removed prior to bond strength testing. (101) Furthermore, microtensile bond strength of porcelain laminate veneer, bonded to enamel after removal of the hypermineralized surface layer, was unaffected by severity of fluorosis. (102) Also, it was reported that shear bond strength was significantly lower with self-etching and etch-and-rinse bonding systems when enamel was ground. (103) It should be remembered that high fluoride concentration is usually in the outer 200µm. (104) This hypermineralized surface layer is more resistant to acid dissolution. Removing the outer 2-3 mm reveals the subsurface enamel, which has a lower fluoride concentration. This may explain why bond strength can be unaffected by the severity of fluorosis when the hypermineralized surface enamel is eliminated.

Studies have indicated that the mode of bond failure is influenced by both age and the severity of fluorosis. Several researchers have examined the bond strength of various bonding systems on fluorosed enamel. Just as in non-fluorosed teeth, bond strength was significantly higher with etch-and-rinse bonding systems than self-etch adhesives.(100) Pre-etching with 37% phosphoric acid improved bonding to moderately and severely fluorosed enamel when self-etching primer was used. (105) The bond strength of 2 mm × 3 mm ceramic discs was investigated (IPS Empress 2) to fluorosed and non-fluorosed tooth surfaces, using etch-and-rinse or self-etch luting resin cements. Shear bond strength was significantly higher with the etch-and-rinse resin cement.(106)

DENTIN

When preparing teeth for laminate veneers or crowns, dentin may occasionally be exposed. Therefore, cementing the restorations with resin cement can involve bonding to dentin. Consequently, understanding the bond strength of resin composite to fluorosed dentin is important. Research found no statistically significant difference in bond strength when using Scotchbond Multipurpose (3M), an etch-and-rinse bonding system, for bonding resin composite to dentin in teeth with mild, moderate, and severe fluorosis. (101) Similarly, it was also observed that fluorosis had no significant effect on shear bond strength when Clearfil SE Bond (Kuraray ESPE) was used as an adhesive. (103) These two studies suggest that fluorosis may not adversely affect adhesive cementation of veneers and crowns to dentin of fluorosed teeth.

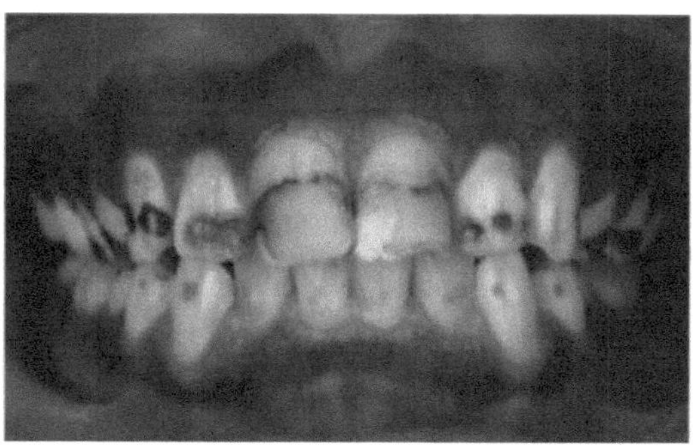

Fig 49: patient with severe dental fluorosis: Pre-operative (source: Lee JD, Inoue N, Lee C, Park S, Lee SJ. Comprehensive Management of Severe Dental Fluorosis with Adhesively Bonded All-Ceramic Restorations. Prosthesis. 2021 Sep;3(3):194–208.

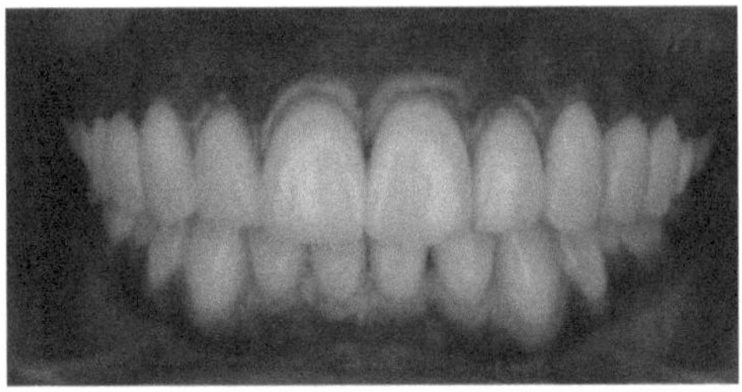

Fig 50: Maxillary and mandibular dentition after final restoration with all ceramic crown. operative (source: Lee JD, Inoue N, Lee C, Park S, Lee SJ. Comprehensive Management of Severe Dental Fluorosis with Adhesively Bonded All-Ceramic Restorations. Prosthesis. 2021 Sep;3(3):194–208.

4) RESIN INFILTRATION TECHNIQUE

The penetration of the resin into the fluorosis lesion is made possible thanks to etching the enamel surface performed with 15% solution of hydrochloric acid for 120 s. This procedure determines the elimination of a 58 μm surface layer of enamel, making accessible the hypomineralized site. Thus, a low-viscosity resin penetrates the porous enamel (108). Fluorotic lesions present with a high degree of subsurface porosity, and these microporosities are filled with either a watery medium or air. Both of these entities have a refractive index (RI) significantly different to that of sound enamel. The differences in refractive indices (RIs) between enamel crystals and the material within the porosities lead to light scattering, causing fluorotic lesions to appear opaque. However, the refractive index of the resin infiltrant is similar to that of sound enamel, so when it penetrates the microporosities, the lesions take on a look similar to the surrounding healthy enamel, as the difference in RIs is negligible. Deeper lesions or those that are already pitted or fissured may require more extensive treatment. Icon is a minimally invasive method that effectively masks fluorotic lesions, with a treatment time shorter than that of micro-abrasion or conventional restorative options, making it particularly advantageous for pediatric patients. Unlike bleaching therapy, which can decrease the microhardness of demineralized enamel surfaces, the resin infiltrant is thought to mechanically strengthen the enamel structure. However, as with tooth whitening and enamel micro-abrasion, the success of resin infiltration is also influenced by the severity of the fluorotic areas. In some cases, only an improvement rather than complete masking of the fluorotic lesion may be achieved.(109)

The commercial infiltration product used is based on triethylene glycol dimethacrylate (TEGDMA). It is necessary for the tooth surface to be mineralized for the resin to infiltrate the enamel via the application of hydrochloric acid. Fluorosis spots already have porous enamel; therefore, the resin can penetrate more easily. Ethanol at a 99% concentration is used to remove water from the pores, facilitating the resin's penetration. The resin must be applied twice because the first application causes contraction of the material as the monomers convert to polymers, resulting in the generation of spaces. The second application must fill these spaces. Resin infiltration proves to be a good option to mask spots associated with mild to moderate fluorosis. Moreover, it is a relatively quick, inexpensive, and minimally invasive treatment.

A young adult with white spot on the upper right central incisor. Application of Icon Etch (15%HCl) for 2 minutes. After rinsing and drying if the white spot is still visible application of Icon Etch should be repeated. After the application of Icon Infiltrant and light-curing for 60 seconds, the spot is well masked. (108)

The concept of deep infiltration involves paying a price in the form of mild mutilation of the enamel through preparation by sandblasting or milling so as to ensure that the infiltration can indeed reach the "ceiling" of the lesion in the case of MIH (Molar incisor hypomineralization) or spread through almost the whole of the lesion if the latter is deep (fluorosis or deep traumatic hypomineralization).(110)
Resin infiltration is found to be the best option in improving esthetics in dental fluorosis. Based on the study done by *Gugnani et al* (111) resin infiltration with additional infiltrant provides the best esthetic result compared with bleaching alone. One of the advantages of resin infiltration is its effectiveness in arresting caries and its application in treating post-orthodontic white spot lesions. Some studies suggest that extending the etching time can enhance the masking of fluorosis stains. The recommended etching duration for the resin infiltration technique is 120 seconds; however, it is primarily advised for active early carious lesions. In the case of fluorosis stains, it may activate inactive lesions. For active caries combined with fluorosis stains, the hypomineralized zone may be deeply seated, making it more resistant to the infiltration process. To ensure proper erosion to the depth of the

hypomineralized zone and subsequent penetration of the infiltrant, the etching of the inactive surface is repeated several times until a visible change in the tooth's color occurs. This etching step can be repeated up to three times, allowing for deeper infiltration and improving the aesthetic outcome.(112)

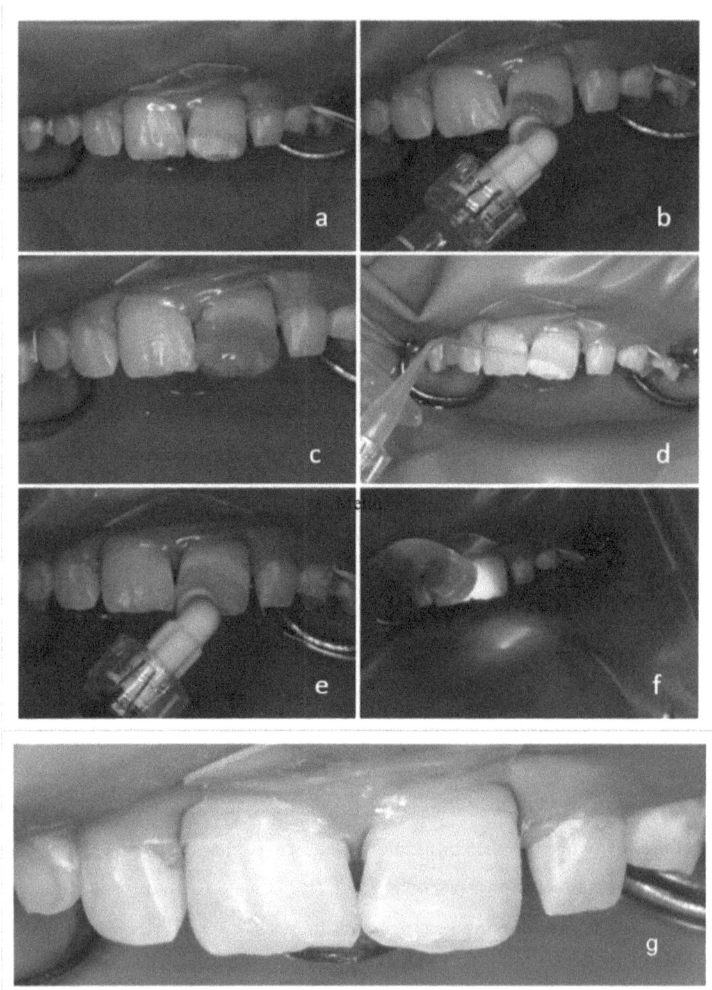

Fig 51: Steps in Icon® application (**a**: Isolation with rubber dam; **b**: Acid application with etch syringe; **c**: Form of the tooth after acid application; **d**: Ethanol application; **e**: Application of resin; **f**: Polymerisation with light); **g**: Clinic photography after post treatment (Source: Clinical evaluation of resin infiltration treatment masking effect on hypomineralised enamel surfaces | BMC Oral Health [cited 2024 Sep 9]. /10.1186/s12903-023-03140-6 (113)

FLUORIDE TOXICITY

Fluoride is widely recognized as an oxidizing agent and a reversible enzymatic inhibitor. It can interfere with the activity of numerous proteins, with at least 80 proteins known to be affected by fluoride.(114)Numerous studies conducted on rodent models have shown that exposure to high levels of fluoride can lead to various metabolic, endocrine, and physiological disorders. Frequent over-exposure to fluoride causes several health problems such as fluorosis, neurological, thyroid, osteoporosis, etc. excessive fluoride exposure may have detrimental effects on overall health. However, it is important to note that the effects of fluoride can depend on factors such as concentration, duration of exposure, and individual susceptibility. Further research is necessary to fully understand the mechanisms and implications of fluoride's inhibitory effects on enzymes and its potential impact on human health.(115) According to a study by *Sharma et al.* fluoride has been associated with neurological damage, which is believed to occur through the mechanisms of oxidative stress and excitotoxicity. Oxidative stress refers to an imbalance between the production of reactive oxygen species (ROS) and the body's ability to neutralize them, leading to cellular damage. In the context of neurodegeneration, oxidative stress can result in the oxidation of essential cellular components such as lipids, proteins, and DNA, ultimately leading to cellular dysfunction and cell death, primarily through apoptosis.

The study suggests that fluoride-induced oxidative stress and excitotoxicity may contribute to neurological damage. Excitotoxicity refers to the harmful overstimulation of neurons, typically caused by excessive activation of receptors for excitatory neurotransmitters such as glutamate. Excitotoxicity can result in the disruption of normal neuronal functioning and potentially contribute to neurodegenerative processes. (116)

The relationship between fluoride exposure, oxidative stress, excitotoxicity, and neurodegeneration requires continued investigation to better assess the potential risks and implications for human health. Children living in areas with high fluoride exposure had lower intelligence quotient (IQ) scores than those living in low-exposure areas. In a cross-sectional study conducted by Sebastian and Sunitha in 2015, it was demonstrated that school children living in areas with high water fluoride levels exhibited more pronounced impairment in intelligence development compared to school children residing in areas with normal or low water fluoride levels. This study suggests that there may be an association between high water fluoride levels and impaired cognitive development in children. However, it's important to note that cross-sectional studies can only establish correlations and cannot determine causation. Further research, including longitudinal studies and controlled trials, is necessary to better understand the potential effects of high fluoride levels on intelligence and cognitive function in children.(117)

It is also worth considering that the impact of fluoride on cognitive development can vary depending on various factors such as the concentration and duration of fluoride exposure, individual susceptibility, and the overall nutritional and environmental context. Thus, additional research is needed to gain a more comprehensive understanding of the relationship between fluoride exposure and cognitive outcomes in children.

In a study conducted by *Peckham et al.* it was found that higher levels of fluoride in drinking water are associated with an increased prevalence of hypothyroidism. The study reported that areas with fluoridated water were nearly twice as likely to have a high prevalence of hypothyroidism compared to non-fluoridated areas. This suggests a potential link between fluoride exposure and thyroid dysfunction.(118) Additionally, *Merdad* found that overweight or obese individuals were more likely to have dental fluorosis compared to those with a healthy weight or underweight. (119) Dental fluorosis is a condition characterized by changes in tooth enamel caused by excessive fluoride intake during tooth development. The study suggests a possible association between obesity and increased susceptibility to dental fluorosis. In a recent study conducted in Russia by *Galkina et al.*,(120) a high prevalence of fluorosis was observed in children and adolescents diagnosed with obesity.

The relationship between fluoride exposure and these health conditions is complex and can be influenced by various factors, including individual susceptibility, overall health status, and the specific characteristics of fluoride exposure.(121)

Most common effects caused by fluoride on the human organism

Fluoride concentration (mg/L)	Effects
0.5–1.0	Improvement of the dental health
1.5–4	Dental fluorosis
> 4	Dental and bone fluorosis
> 10	Degenerative bone fluorosis

Table 12: Revelo-Mejía IA, Hardisson A, Rubio C, Gutiérrez ÁJ, Paz S. Dental Fluorosis: the Risk of Misdiagnosis-a Review. Biol Trace Elem Res. 2021 May;199(5):1762-1770. doi: 10.1007/s12011-020-02296-4. Epub 2020 Jul 23. PMID: 32705431.

Excessive intake of fluoride (F-) can lead to fluorosis. The severity of fluorosis depends on the concentration and frequency of fluoride ingestion. When fluorosis affects the teeth, it is referred to as dental fluorosis. It typically occurs when the concentration of fluoride in drinking water exceeds 1.5 mg/L.

The excessive presence of fluoride in the teeth can interfere with the activity of proteases, which are enzymes involved in protein degradation. This disruption in protease activity can result in abnormal deformation of the enamel structure. Dental pulp cells, specifically ameloblasts (responsible for enamel formation) and odontoblasts (responsible for dentin formation), may undergo decay as a result. These processes contribute to the characteristic effects of dental fluorosis, including discoloration of the teeth and the formation of irregular lesions on the tooth surface. It's important to note that dental fluorosis is a condition that primarily affects the appearance and structure of the teeth. While it may cause cosmetic concerns and mild functional impairment, severe cases of dental fluorosis are relatively rare. The severity of dental fluorosis can vary, ranging from mild white streaks or spots on the enamel to more severe brown discoloration and pitting. [121]

Prevention of dental fluorosis involves monitoring and controlling fluoride intake, particularly in areas where fluoride concentrations in drinking water are elevated. This can be achieved through measures such as community water fluoridation programs and the use of alternative sources of drinking water with lower fluoride levels. Long-term exposure to relatively high levels of fluoride (F-)

at around 4 mg/L can result in skeletal fluorosis, which is another form of fluorosis commonly observed. This occurs when excess fluoride uptake over an extended period leads to its deposition in the bones, causing an increase in bone density. Excessive bone growth may occur in various parts of the body, resulting in skeletal abnormalities and complications such as osteoporosis, paralysis, and neurological disorders (Srivastava and Flora, 2020).

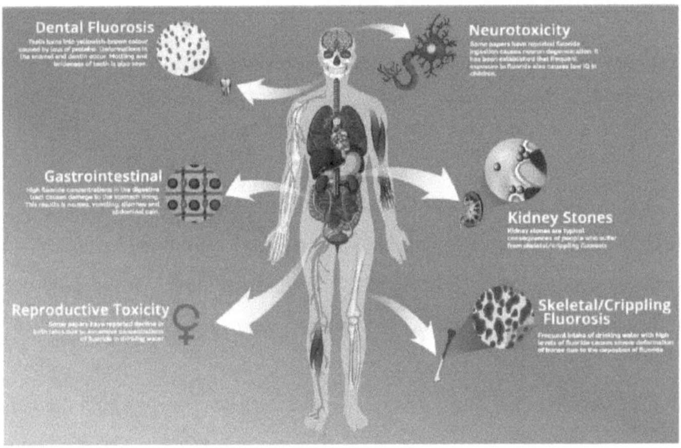

Fig 52 :Adverse health effects on human beings due to ingestion of excess fluoride from drinking water (source: Environmental and Health Effects of Fluoride Contamination and Treatment of Wastewater Using Various Technologies Advanced Treatment Technologies for Fluoride Removal in Water, 2023, Volume 125

Individuals affected by skeletal fluorosis may experience symptoms including muscle weakness, a tingling sensation in the limbs, stiffness in the back, and the formation of abnormal deposits in ligaments. Changes in bone structure and deformities can also be observed. In more severe cases, referred to as crippling fluorosis (usually associated with fluoride levels exceeding 10 mg/L), other organ disorders such as renal (kidney), hepatic (liver), and neuronal (nerve) dysfunction may be present Crippling fluorosis is characterized by significant impairment and can cause severe physical and functional limitations. It is important to note that the prevalence of crippling fluorosis is relatively low, mainly occurring in areas with extremely high fluoride concentrations in drinking water. Prevention and control of skeletal fluorosis involve measures such as ensuring safe and controlled levels of fluoride in drinking water, as well as providing alternative sources of water to areas with high fluoride levels Ingestion of fluoride-contaminated drinking water can lead to gastrointestinal effects, including symptoms such as diarrhea, vomiting, nausea, and abdominal pain. When fluoride (F-) is ingested, it combines with the high acid levels in the stomach and converts into hydrofluoric acid (HF). The disassociation of H+ and F- ions can disrupt enzymatic activity and intracellular pH within cells. The presence of HF in the stomach can cause damage to the stomach lining due to variations in pH. It is worth noting that the severity of gastrointestinal issues is primarily dependent on the aqueous stomach fluoride level rather than the overall amount and regularity of fluoride exposure (Doull et al., 2006). This suggests that even intermittent exposure to high levels of fluoride can lead to gastrointestinal disturbances. In some instances, the consumption of drinking water with high fluoride content has been associated with the development of kidney stones. The exact mechanisms by which fluoride contributes to kidney stone formation are still not fully understood, and further research is needed to establish a clearer understanding of this relationship. [(115)]

To mitigate the risk of gastrointestinal effects and other health issues related to fluoride exposure, it is important to ensure access to safe drinking water sources with appropriate fluoride levels. Monitoring and regulating fluoride concentrations in drinking water supplies are crucial for preventing excessive fluoride ingestion and its associated health implications. Regular monitoring and public health initiatives are necessary to mitigate the risk of excessive fluoride exposure and to address the associated health issues.

CONCLUSION

Fluoride has always been called a double edged sword. On one hand it serves to protect teeth against dental caries and on the other hand it can cause dental fluorosis if consumed in excess and also can lead to not just aesthetic concerns, but also crippling skeletal fluorosis if the consumption is not checked. Due to the increased use of fluoride in preventive dentistry, the prevalence of mild to moderate dental fluorosis is rising in many countries. Effective management strategies typically begin with prevention. However, once the condition has progressed, various treatment options must be considered. The Thylstrup and Fejerskov classification serves as a valuable index for selecting appropriate treatment options for aesthetically concerning fluorosed teeth. In most communities, teeth with a TFI of 3 or higher raise aesthetic concerns, and because the effects on hard dental tissues are irreversible, therapeutic intervention is necessary to enhance their appearance. For cases where more than 50% of surface enamel has been lost (TFI = 8-9), crowning is recommended. However, if a ceramic veneer is bonded to an unprepared tooth surface, fluorosis may compromise bond strength; in such cases, an etch-and-rinse bonding system is preferred. Long-term clinical studies are essential to evaluate the effectiveness of various management options for teeth with differing severities of fluorosis, as measured by TFI.

In summary, there is substantial evidence that fluoridated water, fluoride supplements, infant formulas, and fluoride toothpastes are risk factors for fluorosis, with increasing risk from the use of any one product as the number of products used by the individual increases. Care should be taken when recommending the use of these products in children below the age of six years. Further, the profession needs to make conscious efforts through education to increase the awareness of its members, and of the medical professionals who prescribe the use of these products to patients.

BIBLIOGRAPHY

1. Yadav N, Rani K, Yadav s. s, Yadav DK, Yadav VK, Yadav N. Soil and Water Pollution with Fluoride, Geochemistry, Food Safety Issues and Reclamation-A Review. Int J Curr Microbiol Appl Sci. 2018 May 20;7:1147–62.
2. Goldberg M. Fluoride: Double-Edged Sword Implicated in Caries Prevention and in Fluorosis. J Cell Dev Biol. 2018 Dec 31;1.
3. Soben Peter - Essentials of Public Health Dentistry - WWW - Thedentalhub.org - in PDF | PDF | Dentistry | Dentistry Branches [Internet]. [cited 2024 May 19]. Available from: https://www.scribd.com/document/630008967/soben-peter-Essentials-of-Public-Health-Dentistry-www-thedentalhub-org-in-pdf
4. Ogaard B, Rölla G, Dijkman T, Ruben J, Arends J. Effect of fluoride mouthrinsing on caries lesion development in shark enamel: an in situ caries model study. Scand J Dent Res. 1991 Oct;99(5):372–7.
5. Rošin-Grget K, Peroš K, Sutej I, Bašić K. The cariostatic mechanisms of fluoride. Acta Medica Acad. 2013 Nov;42(2):179–88.
6. Buzalaf MAR, Pessan JP, Honório HM, Ten Cate JM. Mechanisms of action of fluoride for caries control. Monogr Oral Sci. 2011;22:97–114.
7. Groeneveld A, Van Eck AA, Backer Dirks O. Fluoride in caries prevention: is the effect pre- or post-eruptive? J Dent Res. 1990 Feb;69 Spec No:751–5; discussion 820-823.
8. Abanto Alvarez J, Rezende KMPC, Marocho SMS, Alves FBT, Celiberti P, Ciamponi AL. Dental fluorosis: exposure, prevention and management. Med Oral Patol Oral Cirugia Bucal. 2009 Feb 1;14(2):E103-107.
9. Funmilayo AS, Mojirade A. Dental Fluorosis and its Indices, what's new? IOSR J Dent Med Sci. 2014 Jan 1;13:55–60.
10. Akpata ES. Occurrence and management of dental fluorosis. Int Dent J. 2001 Oct;51(5):325–33.
11. DenBesten P, Li W. Chronic fluoride toxicity: dental fluorosis. Monogr Oral Sci. 2011;22:81–96.

12. Gupta N, Gupta N, Chhabra P. Image Diagnosis: Dental and Skeletal Fluorosis. Perm J. 2016;20(1):e105-106.
13. Jha SK, Mishra VK, Sharma DK, Damodaran T. Fluoride in the environment and its metabolism in humans. Rev Environ Contam Toxicol. 2011;211:121–42.
14. Akpata ES. Therapeutic management of dental fluorosis: A critical review of literature. Saudi J Oral Sci. 2014 Jun;1(1):3.
15. Belkhir MS, Douki N. A new concept for removal of dental fluorosis stains. J Endod. 1991 Jun 1;17(6):288–92.
16. Gugnani N, Pandit IK, Gupta M, Gugnani S, Soni S, Goyal V. Comparative evaluation of esthetic changes in nonpitted fluorosis stains when treated with resin infiltration, in-office bleaching, and combination therapies. J Esthet Restor Dent Off Publ Am Acad Esthet Dent Al. 2017 Sep;29(5):317–24.
17. Fluorides in caries prevention | WorldCat.org [Internet]. [cited 2024 Aug 27]. Available from: https://search.worldcat.org/title/Fluorides-in-caries-prevention/oclc/803114715
18. Daly B, Batchelor P, Treasure E. Essential Dental Public Health.
19. Fluoride in Drinking Water: A Scientific Review of EPA's Standards [Internet]. Washington, D.C.: National Academies Press; 2006 [cited 2024 Aug 27]. Available from: http://www.nap.edu/catalog/11571
20. Viswanathan G, Raja PB, Thirumoorthy K, Deepa R, Siva Ilango S. Pathways of factors exacerbating dental fluorosis risk at high altitude regions — A review. Environ Technol Innov. 2020 Nov 1;20:101115.
21. McDonagh MS, Whiting PF, Wilson PM, Sutton AJ, Chestnutt I, Cooper J, et al. Systematic review of water fluoridation. BMJ. 2000 Oct 7;321(7265):855–9.
22. Kallala R, Slimani A, Gassara Y, Garrach B, Chouchen S, Foddha H, et al. The association between Dental Fluorosis and COL1A2 gene polymorphism among a Tunisian Population. BMC Oral Health. 2024 Mar 22;24:376.
23. Irigoyen-Camacho ME, García Pérez A, Mejía González A, Huizar Alvarez R. Nutritional status and dental fluorosis among schoolchildren in communities with different drinking water fluoride concentrations in a central region in Mexico. Sci Total Environ. 2016 Jan 15;541:512–9.

24. Morgan L, Allred E, Tavares M, Bellinger D, Needleman H. Investigation of the possible associations between fluorosis, fluoride exposure, and childhood behavior problems. Pediatr Dent. 1998;20(4):244–52.
25. Arends J, Christoffersen J. Nature and role of loosely bound fluoride in dental caries. J Dent Res. 1990 Feb;69 Spec No:601–5; discussion 634-636.
26. Featherstone JD. Prevention and reversal of dental caries: role of low level fluoride. Community Dent Oral Epidemiol. 1999 Feb;27(1):31–40.
27. Rølla G. On the role of calcium fluoride in the cariostatic mechanism of fluoride. Acta Odontol Scand. 1988 Dec;46(6):341–5.
28. Chemical interactions between the tooth and oral fluids | Request PDF [Internet]. [cited 2024 May 19]. Available from: https://www.researchgate.net/publication/289638326_Chemical_interactions_between_the_tooth_and_oral_fluids
29. Koo H. Strategies to enhance the biological effects of fluoride on dental biofilms. Adv Dent Res. 2008 Jul 1;20(1):17–21.
30. Ekstrand J, Oliveby A. Fluoride in the oral environment. Acta Odontol Scand. 1999 Dec;57(6):330–3.
31. Oliveby A, Ekstrand J, Lagerlöf F. Effect of salivary flow rate on salivary fluoride clearance after use of a fluoride-containing chewing gum. Caries Res. 1987;21(5):393–401.
32. Oliveby A, Twetman S, Ekstrand J. Diurnal fluoride concentration in whole saliva in children living in a high- and a low-fluoride area. Caries Res. 1990;24(1):44–7.
33. Tatevossian A. Fluoride in dental plaque and its effects. J Dent Res. 1990 Feb;69 Spec No:645–52; discussion 682-683.
34. Ekstrand J. Fluoride in plaque fluid and saliva after NaF or MFP rinses. Eur J Oral Sci. 1997 Oct;105(5 Pt 2):478–84.
35. Dawes C, Weatherell JA. Kinetics of fluoride in the oral fluids. J Dent Res. 1990 Feb;69 Spec No:638–44; discussion 682-683.
36. Whitford GM. Intake and metabolism of fluoride. Adv Dent Res. 1994 Jun;8(1):5–14.
37. Weatherell JA, Robinson C, Hallsworth AS. Changes in the fluoride concentration of the labial enamel surface with age. Caries Res. 1972;6(4):312–24.

38. Nakagaki H, Koyama Y, Sakakibara Y, Weatherell JA, Robinson C. Distribution of fluoride across human dental enamel, dentine and cementum. Arch Oral Biol. 1987;32(9):651–4.
39. dokumen.pub [Internet]. [cited 2024 May 19]. Orban's Oral Histology & Embryology [15 ed.] 9788131254820, 8131254828. Available from: https://dokumen.pub/orbans-oral-histology-amp-embryology-15nbsped-9788131254820-8131254828.html
40. Singer L, Armstrong WD. Comparison of Fluoride Contents of Human Dental and Skeletal Tissues. J Dent Res. 1962 Jan 1;41(1):154–7.
41. Hallsworth AS, Weatherell JA. The microdistribution, uptake and loss of fluoride in human enamel. Caries Res. 1969;3(2):109–18.
42. Vieira APGF, Hancock R, Dumitriu M, Limeback H, Grynpas MD. Fluoride's effect on human dentin ultrasound velocity (elastic modulus) and tubule size. Eur J Oral Sci. 2006 Feb;114(1):83–8.
43. Primary tooth fluorosis and fluoride intake during the first year of life - PubMed [Internet]. [cited 2024 Sep 4]. Available from: https://pubmed.ncbi.nlm.nih.gov/12147170/
44. Michel-Crosato E, Biazevic MGH, Crosato E. Relationship between dental fluorosis and quality of life: a population based study. Braz Oral Res. 2005;19(2):150–5.
45. Srivastava R, Tangade P, Priyadarshi S. Managing dental fluorosis: A guide to improving appearance of the teeth. Arch Dent Res. 13(1):25–9.
46. Smith CE, Nanci A, Denbesten PK. Effects of chronic fluoride exposure on morphometric parameters defining the stages of amelogenesis and ameloblast modulation in rat incisors. Anat Rec. 1993 Oct;237(2):243–58.
47. Kierdorf H, Kierdorf U. Disturbances of the secretory stage of amelogenesis in fluorosed deer teeth: a scanning electron-microscopic study. Cell Tissue Res. 1997 Jul;289(1):125–35.
48. Bronckers ALJJ, Lyaruu DM, Bervoets TJM, Wöltgens JHM. Fluoride enhances intracellular degradation of amelogenins during secretory phase of amelogenesis of hamster teeth in organ culture. Connect Tissue Res. 2002;43(2–3):456–65.
49. Den Besten PK. Effects of fluoride on protein secretion and removal during enamel development in the rat. J Dent Res. 1986 Oct;65(10):1272–7.

50. Suckling G, Thurley DC, Nelson DG. The macroscopic and scanning electron-microscopic appearance and microhardness of the enamel, and the related histological changes in the enamel organ of erupting sheep incisors resulting from a prolonged low daily dose of fluoride. Arch Oral Biol. 1988;33(5):361–73.
51. Bronckers AL, Jansen LL, Wöltgens JH. Long-term (8 days) effects of exposure to low concentrations of fluoride on enamel formation in hamster tooth-germs in organ culture in vitro. Arch Oral Biol. 1984;29(10):811–9.
52. Zhou R, Zaki AE, Eisenmann DR. Morphometry and autoradiography of altered rat enamel protein processing due to chronic exposure to fluoride. Arch Oral Biol. 1996;41(8–9):739–47.
53. Denbesten PK, Crenshaw MA, Wilson MH. Changes in the fluoride-induced modulation of maturation stage ameloblasts of rats. J Dent Res. 1985 Dec;64(12):1365–70.
54. Variations in the composition of developing rat incisor enamel - PubMed [Internet]. [cited 2024 Sep 4]. Available from: https://pubmed.ncbi.nlm.nih.gov/1148889/
55. Ja W, D D, C R, As H. Fluoride concentrations in developing enamel. Nature [Internet]. 1975 Jul 17 [cited 2024 Sep 4];256(5514). Available from: https://pubmed.ncbi.nlm.nih.gov/1152994/
56. DenBesten PK, Thariani H. Biological mechanisms of fluorosis and level and timing of systemic exposure to fluoride with respect to fluorosis. J Dent Res. 1992 May;71(5):1238–43.
57. Crenshaw MA, Bawden JW. Fluoride-binding by organic matrix from early and late developing bovine fetal enamel determined by flow-rate dialysis. Arch Oral Biol. 1981 Jan 1;26(6):473–6.
58. Robinson C, Kirkham J. The effect of fluoride on the developing mineralized tissues. J Dent Res. 1990 Feb;69 Spec No:685–91; discussion 721.
59. DenBesten PK. Biological mechanisms of dental fluorosis relevant to the use of fluoride supplements. Community Dent Oral Epidemiol. 1999 Feb;27(1):41–7.
60. DenBesten PK, Heffernan LM. Enamel proteases in secretory and maturation enamel of rats ingesting 0 and 100 PPM fluoride in drinking water. Adv Dent Res. 1989 Sep;3(2):199–202.

61. Ramesh M, Narasimhan M, Krishnan R, Aruna RM, Kuruvilla S. The effect of fluorosis on human teeth under light microscopy: A cross-sectional study. J Oral Maxillofac Pathol JOMFP. 2017;21(3):345–50.
62. Fejerskov O, Johnson NW, Silverstone LM. The ultrastructure of fluorosed human dental enamel. Scand J Dent Res. 1974;82(5):357–72.
63. Robinson C, Connell S, Kirkham J, Brookes SJ, Shore RC, Smith AM. The effect of fluoride on the developing tooth. Caries Res. 2004;38(3):268–76.
64. Fejerskov O, Manji F, Baelum V. The nature and mechanisms of dental fluorosis in man. J Dent Res. 1990 Feb;69 Spec No:692–700; discussion 721.
65. Susheela: Structural aberrations in fluorosed human... - Google Scholar [Internet]. [cited 2024 Sep 5]. Available from: https://scholar.google.com/scholar_lookup?journal=Current+Sci&title=Structural+aberrations+in+fluorosed+human+teeth:+Biochemical+and+scanning+electron+microscopic+studies&author=AK+Susheela&author=M+Bhatnagar&volume=77&publication_year=1999&pages=1-6&
66. Thylstrup A, Fejerskov O. Clinical appearance of dental fluorosis in permanent teeth in relation to histologic changes. Community Dent Oral Epidemiol. 1978 Nov;6(6):315–28.
67. Priyadharsini N, Malathi N, Tamizhchelvan H, Dineshkumar T. Dental fluorosis: A histological study using Light and Confocal microscopy. Indian J Dent Res Off Publ Indian Soc Dent Res. 2015;26(3):248–51.
68. Pizzo G, Piscopo MR, Pizzo I, Giuliana G. Community water fluoridation and caries prevention: a critical review. Clin Oral Investig. 2007 Sep;11(3):189–93.
69. (PDF) Fluoride Toxicity: A Review on Dental Fluorosis and Its Prevalence in India [Internet]. [cited 2024 Sep 2]. Available from: https://www.researchgate.net/publication/339458489_Fluoride_Toxicity_A_Review_on_Dental_Fluorosis_and_Its_Prevalence_in_India
70. Dwivedi S, Dwivedi N. Environmental aspects of fluoride contamination and treatment of wastewater using hybrid technology. In 2021. p. 445–61.
71. Patterns of Dental Fluorosis in a European Country in Relation to the Fluoride Concentration of Drinking Water - M.J. Larsen, E. Kirkegaard, S. Poulsen, 1987 [Internet]. [cited 2024 Sep 5]. Available from: https://journals.sagepub.com/doi/abs/10.1177/00220345870660010101

72. (PDF) Prevalence, severity and factors associated with dental fluorosis among children aged 8-10 years in Bangkok, Thailand [Internet]. [cited 2024 Sep 11]. Available from: https://www.researchgate.net/publication/310440655_Prevalence_severity_and_factors_associated_with_dental_fluorosis_among_children_aged_8-10_years_in_Bangkok_Thailand
73. Cutress TW, Suckling GW. Differential diagnosis of dental fluorosis. J Dent Res. 1990 Feb;69 Spec No:714–20; discussion 721.
74. Dental fluorosis in Australia [Internet]. Fluoride Free Australia. 2018 [cited 2024 Sep 11]. Available from: https://fluoridefreeaustralia.org/dental-fluorosis/
75. Choubisa S. Status of chronic fluoride exposure and its adverse health consequences in the tribal people of the scheduled area of Rajasthan, India. 2022 Jun 18;55:8–30.
76. Hattab FN, Qudeimat MA, al-Rimawi HS. Dental discoloration: an overview. J Esthet Dent. 1999;11(6):291–310.
77. L STK, Shetty S, M AB, Pujari SC, P SR, Nandlal B. A Pioneering Study of Dental Fluorosis in the Libyan Population. J Int Oral Health JIOH. 2013 Jun;5(3):67–72.
78. Patidar D, Sogi S, Patidar D, Sharma A, Jain M, Prasad P. Enlightening Diagnosis and Differential Diagnosis of Dental Fluorosis—A Hidden Entity in a Crowd. Dent J Adv Stud. 2021 Mar 18;9.
79. Thylstrup A. Distribution of dental fluorosis in the primary dentition. Community Dent Oral Epidemiol. 1978 Nov;6(6):329–37.
80. Mohd Nor NA. Methods and indices in measuring fluorosis: A review. Arch Orofac Sci. 2017 Dec 1;12:77–85.
81. Dean HT. Classification of Mottled Enamel Diagnosis. J Am Dent Assoc 1922. 1934 Aug 1;21(8):1421–6.
82. Riordan PJ, Banks JA. Dental fluorosis and fluoride exposure in Western Australia. J Dent Res. 1991 Jul;70(7):1022–8.
83. Granath L, Widenheim J, Birkhed D. Diagnosis of mild enamel fluorosis in permanent maxillary incisors using two scoring systems. Community Dent Oral Epidemiol. 1985 Oct;13(5):273–6.

84. Horowitz HS, Driscoll WS, Meyers RJ, Heifetz SB, Kingman A. A new method for assessing the prevalence of dental fluorosis--the Tooth Surface Index of Fluorosis. J Am Dent Assoc 1939. 1984 Jul;109(1):37–41.
85. Pendrys DG. The fluorosis risk index: a method for investigating risk factors. J Public Health Dent. 1990;50(5):291–8.
86. Clarkson J, O'Mullane D. A modified DDE Index for use in epidemiological studies of enamel defects. J Dent Res. 1989 Mar;68(3):445–50.
87. (PDF) Prevalence of Enamel Defects in Permanent Teeth of Patients With Complete Cleft Lip and Palate [Internet]. [cited 2024 Sep 1]. Available from: https://www.researchgate.net/publication/221794064_Prevalence_of_Enamel_Defects_in_Permanent_Teeth_of_Patients_With_Complete_Cleft_Lip_and_Palate
88. (PDF) Developmental Defects of Enamel : an increasing reality in the everyday practice [Internet]. [cited 2024 Sep 1]. Available from: https://www.researchgate.net/publication/269687998_Developmental_Defects_of_Enamel_an_increasing_reality_in_the_everyday_practice
89. Khyalia P, Jugiani H, Dangi J, Laura J, Nandal M. A Comprehensive Review on the Techniques and Indexes Used for the Analysis of Fluorosis in Humans and Cattle. Orient J Chem. 2023 Oct 31;39:1120–32.
90. Goyal A, Verma M, Toteja G, Gauba K, Mohanty V, Mohanty U, et al. Validation of ICMR index for identification of dental fluorosis in epidemiological studies. Indian J Med Res. 2016;144(1):52.
91. Guidelines for drinking-water quality, 1st edition: Volume 1 - Recommendations [Internet]. [cited 2024 Sep 9]. Available from: https://www.who.int/publications/i/item/9241541687
92. Ophaug RH, Singer L, Harland BF. Dietary fluoride intake of 6-month and 2-year-old children in four dietary regions of the United States. Am J Clin Nutr. 1985 Oct;42(4):701–7.
93. Bentley EM, Ellwood RP, Davies RM. Fluoride ingestion from toothpaste by young children. Br Dent J. 1999 May 8;186(9):460–2.
94. Bussadori SK, do Rego MA, da Silva PE, Pinto MM, Pinto ACG. Esthetic alternative for fluorosis blemishes with the usage of a dual bleaching system based on hydrogen peroxide at 35%. J Clin Pediatr Dent. 2004;28(2):143–6.

95. Wright JT. The etch-bleach-seal technique for managing stained enamel defects in young permanent incisors. Pediatr Dent. 2002;24(3):249–52.
96. Katarmal DB. Dental Bleaching for Fluorosis of Teeth [Internet]. [cited 2024 Sep 6]. Available from: https://www.drkatarmal.com/2014/12/dental-bleaching-for-fluorosis-of-teeth.html
97. DenBesten PK, Thariani H. Biological mechanisms of fluorosis and level and timing of systemic exposure to fluoride with respect to fluorosis. J Dent Res. 1992 May;71(5):1238–43.
98. Christensen GJ. Clinical factors affecting adhesion. Oper Dent. 1992;Suppl 5:24–31.
99. Al-Sugair MH, Akpata ES. Effect of fluorosis on etching of human enamel. J Oral Rehabil. 1999 Jun;26(6):521–8.
100. Ertuğrul F, Türkün M, Türkün LS, Toman M, Cal E. Bond strength of different dentin bonding systems to fluorotic enamel. J Adhes Dent. 2009 Aug;11(4):299–303.
101. Ateyah N, Akpata E. Factors affecting shear bond strength of composite resin to fluorosed human enamel. Oper Dent. 2000;25(3):216–22.
102. Ratnaweera PM, Fukagawa N, Tsubota Y, Fukushima S. Microtensile bond strength of porcelain laminate veneers bonded to fluorosed teeth. J Prosthodont Off J Am Coll Prosthodont. 2009 Apr;18(3):205–10.
103. Ermis RB, De Munck J, Cardoso MV, Coutinho E, Van Landuyt KL, Poitevin A, et al. Bonding to ground versus unground enamel in fluorosed teeth. Dent Mater Off Publ Acad Dent Mater. 2007 Oct;23(10):1250–5.
104. Richards A, Fejerskov O, Baelum V. Enamel fluoride in relation to severity of human dental fluorosis. Adv Dent Res. 1989 Sep;3(2):147–53.
105. Weerasinghe DS, Nikaido T, Wettasinghe KA, Abayakoon JB, Tagami J. Micro-shear bond strength and morphological analysis of a self-etching primer adhesive system to fluorosed enamel. J Dent. 2005 May;33(5):419–26.
106. Toman M, Cal E, Türkün M, Ertuğrul F. Bond strength of glass-ceramics on the fluorosed enamel surfaces. J Dent. 2008 Apr;36(4):281–6.
107. Lee JD, Inoue N, Lee C, Park S, Lee SJ. Comprehensive Management of Severe Dental Fluorosis with Adhesively Bonded All-Ceramic Restorations. Prosthesis. 2021 Sep;3(3):194–208.

108. Zotti F, Albertini L, Tomizioli N, Capocasale G, Albanese M. Resin Infiltration in Dental Fluorosis Treatment—1-Year Follow-Up. Medicina (Mex). 2020 Dec 29;57(1):22.
109. Muñoz MA, Arana-Gordillo LA, Gomes GM, Gomes OM, Bombarda NHC, Reis A, et al. Alternative esthetic management of fluorosis and hypoplasia stains: blending effect obtained with resin infiltration techniques. J Esthet Restor Dent Off Publ Am Acad Esthet Dent Al. 2013 Feb;25(1):32–9.
110. Treatment of Fluorosis Spots Using a Resin Infiltration Technique: 14-month Follow-up - PubMed [Internet]. [cited 2024 Sep 6]. Available from: https://pubmed.ncbi.nlm.nih.gov/27455116/
111. Gugnani N, Pandit IK, Goyal V, Gugnani S, Sharma J, Dogra S. Esthetic improvement of white spot lesions and non-pitted fluorosis using resin infiltration technique: series of four clinical cases. J Indian Soc Pedod Prev Dent. 2014;32(2):176–80.
112. Shahroom NSB, Mani G, Ramakrishnan M. Interventions in management of dental fluorosis, an endemic disease: A systematic review. J Fam Med Prim Care. 2019 Oct 31;8(10):3108–13.
113. Clinical evaluation of resin infiltration treatment masking effect on hypomineralised enamel surfaces | BMC Oral Health | Full Text [Internet]. [cited 2024 Sep 9]. Available from: https://bmcoralhealth.biomedcentral.com/articles/10.1186/s12903-023-03140-6
114. García-Montalvo EA, Reyes-Pérez H, Del Razo LM. Fluoride exposure impairs glucose tolerance via decreased insulin expression and oxidative stress. Toxicology. 2009 Sep 19;263(2–3):75–83.
115. (PDF) Fluoride Interactions: From Molecules to Disease [Internet]. [cited 2024 May 19]. Available from: https://www.researchgate.net/publication/233517970_Fluoride_Interactions_From_Molecules_to_Disease
116. Sharma C, Suhalka P, Sukhwal P, Jaiswal N, Bhatnagar M. Curcumin attenuates neurotoxicity induced by fluoride: An in vivo evidence. Pharmacogn Mag. 2014 Jan;10(37):61–5.

117. A cross-sectional study to assess the intelligence quotient (IQ) of school going children aged 10-12 years in villages of Mysore district, India with different fluoride levels - PubMed [Internet]. [cited 2024 May 19]. Available from: https://pubmed.ncbi.nlm.nih.gov/26381633/
118. Peckham S, Lowery D, Spencer S. Are fluoride levels in drinking water associated with hypothyroidism prevalence in England? A large observational study of GP practice data and fluoride levels in drinking water. J Epidemiol Community Health. 2015 Jul;69(7):619–24.
119. MERDAD HE. Predicting Dental Fluorosis Using Indicators of Childhood Obesity. In 2013.
120. Galkina IV, Gavrilova OA, Piekalnits II, Dianov OA. [Dental status in children and adolescents diagnosed with obesity]. Stomatologiia (Sofiia). 2015;94(1):57–8.
121. Revelo-Mejía IA, Hardisson A, Rubio C, Gutiérrez ÁJ, Paz S. Dental Fluorosis: the Risk of Misdiagnosis-a Review. Biol Trace Elem Res. 2021 May;199(5):1762–70.

TABLE OF CONTENTS

INTRODUCTION	1
HISTORY	7
ETIOLOGY	11
MECHANISM OF ACTION OF FLUORIDE	20
DISTRIBUTION OF FLUORIDE IN ORAL CAVITY	26
PATHOPHYSIOLOGY	30
HISTOPATHOLOGY	36
CLINICAL FEATURES	45
DIFFERENTIAL DIAGNOSIS OF FLUOROSIS	51
DIAGNOSIS	57
INDICES	62
MANAGEMENT OF FLUROSIS	77
FLUORIDE TOXICITY	93
CONCLUSION	98
BIBLIOGRAPHY	99

FSC
www.fsc.org
MIX
Papier | Fördert
gute Waldnutzung
FSC® C083411

Kolibri 360 GmbH
Ferdinand-Jühlke-Straße 7
99095 Erfurt, Deutschland
produktsicherheit@kolibri360.de

Druck:
CPI Druckdienstleistungen GmbH
im Auftrag der
Kolibri 360 GmbH
Ferdinand-Jühlke-Str. 7
99095 Erfurt